George Murray Humphry

Old Age

The Results of Information Received Respecting nearly Nine Hundred Persons who

Had Attained the Age of Eighty Years

George Murray Humphry

Old Age

*The Results of Information Received Respecting nearly Nine Hundred Persons who Had
Attained the Age of Eighty Years*

ISBN/EAN: 9783337306793

Printed in Europe, USA, Canada, Australia, Japan

Cover: Foto ©Suzi / pixelio.de

More available books at **www.hansebooks.com**

OLD AGE,

THE RESULTS OF INFORMATION RECEIVED RESPECTING
NEARLY NINE HUNDRED PERSONS WHO HAD
ATTAINED THE AGE OF EIGHTY YEARS,
INCLUDING SEVENTY-FOUR CENTENARIANS.

BY

GEORGE MURRAY HUMPHRY, M.D., F.R.S.,

FELLOW OF KING'S COLLEGE, HON. FELLOW OF DOWNING COLLEGE,
PROFESSOR OF SURGERY IN THE UNIVERSITY OF CAMBRIDGE,
AND SURGEON TO ADDENBROOKE'S HOSPITAL.

CAMBRIDGE:
MACMILLAN AND BOWES.
1889

PREFACE.

In my Presidential Address at the Cambridge Meeting of the British Medical Association in 1880 I drew attention to the advantages that might be derived by utilizing the organisation of that great body, then numbering more than eight thousand members (it now numbers about thirteen thousand), for the purpose of collecting information upon various subjects of medical interest. A "Collective Investigation Committee" was consequently formed, and carefully-considered Circulars of Inquiry upon several subjects were issued. The replies were tabulated and analysed, and reports and memoranda upon them were issued, from time to time, in the *Collective Investigation Record* and in the *British Medical Journal*, as follows : On the Communicability of Phthisis, by Dr Burney Yeo ; On Acute Pneumonia, by Drs Sturges and Sidney Coupland, with appendices by Surgeon-major Maunsell and Drs Finlayson, Longstaff, and Giles ; On Chorea, by Dr Stephen Mackenzie ; On Acute Rheumatism, by Dr Whipham (a Preliminary Report by Dr Mahomed) ; On Diphtheria, by Mr Shirley Murphy ; On Puerperal Pyrexia, by Dr Galabin and Mr Oswald Browne ; On Acute Gout, by Sir Dyce Duckworth ; On Cancer of the Breast, by Mr Butlin ; On Old Age, on Centenarians, on the Maladies of Old People, and on Aged Persons, by myself; On the Connection of Disease with Habits of Intemperance, and on the Geographical Distribution of Certain Diseases in the British Islands (with Maps), by Dr Isambard Owen; and On the Causes of Death among Gouty Men, by Dr Edward Casey.

The labour attendant upon the work, it need scarcely be said, has been great, and the expense, the funds for defraying which have been liberally supplied by the Association, has been considerable. The onerous office of Secretary to the Committee was first held by Dr Mahomed. At his death, when a promising career was cut short by one of those contagious attacks from which the public erroneously imagines that medical men enjoy a sort of charmed exemption, Dr Herringham and, subsequently, Dr Isambard Owen were good enough to undertake the work; and it is to the energy, good judgment and ability of these gentlemen that the success of the movement has been mainly due.

The following Inquiry-Paper was issued concerning the general condition, habits, and circumstances, past and present, and the Family History of PERSONS who had attained or passed the AGE of EIGHTY YEARS; and directions were given as to the manner in which the replies should be made.

CONDITION AT THE PRESENT TIME.

Name or Initials.
Age. Male or female. Single, married, widowed.
Residence. Occupation.
Circumstances.—Affluent, comfortable, poor.

GENERAL CONDITION.

Fat, spare, average; full-blooded, pale, average; strong, feeble, average.

Height feet inches. *Weight* . *Figure.*—Erect, bent.

VOICE.—Loud, clear, full, weak.

SIGHT.—Good, short, long. Are glasses required for reading? If so, for how many years?

HEARING.—Good, bad, indifferent.

Are the joints of the fingers or hands natural, stiff, or deformed?

TEETH.—How many remaining? Artificial teeth used? If so, how long?

DIGESTION.—Good, bad, moderate.

Appetite.—Good, bad, moderate.

Small eater, large eater, moderate. How many meals each day?

Amount and kind of alcoholic beverages daily?

    „   „   other beverages daily?

Amount of animal food daily?

Bowels.—Act daily, alternate days, irregularly. Are aperient medicines taken frequently or rarely?

DISPOSITION.—Placid, irritable, energetic, lethargic.

INTELLECTUAL POWERS.—High, low, average. Give any details.

Memory.—Good, bad, moderate, for past or recent events.

HABITS.—Active, sedentary, confined to bed. Amount and kind of out-door exercise.

Smokes tobacco.—Much, little, moderately. *Takes snuff.*

Sleep.—Good, bad, moderate. No. of hours . Hour of going to bed . Of rising .

ANY PRESENT MALADIES.—Their nature and duration.

State any other points in the general condition, habits, etc., worthy of mention.

PAST HISTORY.

Occupation.

Residences.

Age when married. Duration of married life. No. of children.

Circumstances.—Affluent, comfortable, poor.

First, second, third, or child of parents.

GENERAL CONDITION.—Stout, spare, average; delicate, robust, average; health usually good, moderate, often ailing, rarely ailing.

DIGESTION.—Usually good, indifferent.

H. C.   *b*

Bowels.—Usual condition of.

Baldness or *greyness* of hair; occurring early in life, or late.

DISPOSITION.—Placid, irritable, energetic, lethargic.

INTELLECTUAL POWERS.—High, low, average. Any special evidence respecting them.

HABITS.—Active, sedentary, moderate. Amount and kind of out-door exercise.

    Hours in bed   , hour of rising   .

    Good, bad, average sleeper.

APPETITE.—Good, indifferent. Large, small, average eater.

    Amount and kind of alcoholic beverages daily.

    ,,   ,,   other beverages daily.

    Amount of animal food daily.

Smoked tobacco.—Much, little, moderately.   *Has taken snuff.*

ILLNESSES UNDERGONE.—Their nature, and the period at which they occurred. Whether severe. Their duration and the completeness of recovery.

SLIGHT AILMENTS.—To which specially liable; and period of life at which they occurred.

ACCIDENTS.—With dates.

State any other points or peculiarities which may seem worthy of mention, in the case of either sex.

FAMILY HISTORY.

AGE AT DEATH and CAUSE OF DEATH.—Of Father's Father; of Father's Mother; of Mother's Father; of Mother's Mother; of Father; of Mother; of Brothers; of Sisters; of Sons; of Daughters.

Ages of brothers now alive; of sisters; of children.

Was there any, and if any, what, blood-relationship between father and mother, or between grandparents on either side?

Age of Father when the subject of the inquiry was born; do. of Mother.

Is any member of the family known to have had cancer, consumption, scrofula, gout, rheumatism, epilepsy, or insanity? State which member in each case.

State any other points in family history that may seem worthy of mention.

THE FOLLOWING QUESTIONS CAN ONLY BE ANSWERED BY A MEDICAL MAN.

    CHEST-GIRTH round nipples in inspiration, number of inches; do. in expiration.

ELASTICITY of rib-cartilages (*as ascertained by gentle pressure upon them, and upon lower end of sternum*), distinct, indistinct.

PULSE.—No. per minute, regular, intermitting, large, small, compressible, incompressible.

ARTERIES.—Tortuous, visible, even, knotty.

RESPIRATIONS.—No. per minute, regular, irregular.

ARCUS SENILIS.—Much, little, absent.

TEETH.—How many remaining?

Upper incisors ; canine ; molar ;

Lower   ,, ; ,, ; ,,

ANY EVIDENCE OF FAILURE of heart, lungs, brain, urinary or other organs?

MICTURITION.—Slow, difficult, painful, natural.

Nearly nine hundred returns were received and forwarded to me, and were tabulated and analysed; and the results, representing as may be supposed no small amount of labour, were published in the *British Medical Journal* and the *Collective Investigation Record*, and, with the sanction of the Committee, are republished, with some additions, in the present little volume.

There are many points upon which additional information is to be desired, and room is left for further investigation; but so large an amount of material relating to the subject of OLD AGE has, I suppose, never been collected before. I have often wished that the opportunity of dealing with it had fallen into abler hands; but I doubt whether any one would have bestowed more pains upon it than I have done, and my thanks are due to the many persons who have assisted in the inquiry.

The medical men who were good enough to make returns, and the number of returns made by each, are as follows—

Airy, Dr (1); Alderson, T., Hammersmith (11); Allan, Dr, Leeds (6); Alliott, Dr, Sevenoaks (2); Atkinson, Dr, Surbiton (3); Arnold, C. Aberdeen (2); Barker, Dr, Sandown (2); Barnes, Dr, Carlisle (3);

Barnes, J., Clare (1); Barnes, Dr, Eye (8); Barron, Mr, Durham (1);
Batterbury, Dr, Berkhamsted (2); Beale, Dr, London (4); Bell, Dr,
Eastbourne (1); Berry, Dr, Watford (5); Berry, W., Wigan (3); Beverley,
Dr, Norwich (5); Black, J., London (1); Blair, Dr, Shotts (5); Booth,
D, Aberdeen (1); Booth, Dr, Durham (4); Bowles, Dr, Folkestone (5);
Boyce, C., Maidstone (2); Bradford, E., Harrow (1); Brett, Dr, Wat-
ford (6); Braidwood, Dr, Birkenhead (2); Bridger, Dr, Cottenham (4);
Briscoe, J., London (2); Bumpsted, T., Cambridge (1); Burd, Dr,
Shrewsbury (25); Burrows, Sir G., London (1); Burton, W., Thornton
(1); Burry, Dr, Liphook (1); Burry, G., Whetstone (1); Caldwell, J.,
Shotts (2); Camphill, Dr, Liverpool (1); Carver, E., Cambridge (1);
Casey, Dr, Windsor (4); Chevalier, Dr, Ipswich (3); Clarke, F., Bury
St Edmunds (1); Clutton, H., London (1); Coghill, Dr, Ventnor (1);
Colman, Dr, Kensington (2); Copley, Mr, Wisbech (2); Cory, Dr,
London (2); Coxwell, Dr, (1); Crallan, Dr, Fulbourne (3); Cribb, Dr,
London (2); Crombie, J., Brentford (1); Cronier, H., Jersey (1); Cross-
man, Mr, Hambrook (3); Crowe, Dr, Worcester (1); Cullimore, Dr,
London (1); Dall, J., Newcastle (4); Davies-Colley, N., London (1);
Davis, Dr, London (26); De Ville, Dr, Harrogate (2); Donald T.,
Kingston-on-Thames (1); Douglas, Dr, Newbury (2); Drummond, J.,
Shields (1); Duckworth, Sir Dyce, London (2); Duncan, W., Ottery (3);
Dunlop, Dr, Jersey (3); Eastes, Dr, London (1); Eddowes, A., Market
Drayton (1); Edwards, G. C., Ipswich (1); Emerson, P., Southwold (2);
Esler, Dr, Belfast (10); Ewart, Dr, London (1); Ferris, Dr, Uxbridge (1);
Fielding, Dr, Milton Abbas (2); Finlay, Dr, London (3); Fisher, Dr,
Brighton (1); Fleming, Dr, Glasgow (1); Fletcher, Dr, Ormskirk (1);
Frazer, Dr, Bournemouth (1); Forty, Dr, Wotton-under-Edge (1); Fox,
H. C., Stoke Newington (3); Galton, J. H., London (3); Galton, Dr,
London (2); George, H., Louth (1); Giddings, Dr, Leeds (1); Gilbert,
E., Amherst (1); Gilmour, Dr, Glasgow (1); Godfrey, Dr, St Heliers (3);
Gorham, J., Galway (2); Graham, Dr, Weybridge (6); Gray, C., New-
market (1); Grant, Dr, Inverness (1); Green, T. B., Kendal (1); Green,
J., Salisbury (7); Green, W., Sandown (5); Gripper, Dr, Wallington (1);
Groom, Dr, Wisbech (3); Gross, C., Walworth (2); Ground, E., Maidstone
(1); Hall, W., Lancaster (3); Hammond, Dr, Nuneaton (1); Hannah,
Mr, Ashton (5); Harrison, Dr, Huddersfield (5); Harris, Dr, London (1);
Harvey, F., Plymouth Hospital (1); Hayman, S., Abington (2); Hay-
ward, J., Whitstable (3); Head, Dr, Carlisle (1); Heysham, Mr, Win-
chester (1); Hills, T. Hyde, Cambridge (2); Hodson, C., Bishop's
Stortford (1); Holden, Dr, Sudbury (3); Hollis, Dr, Brighton (1); Hol-
man, H., Hothly (2); Hovell, D., Elstree (1); Humphry, Professor,

Cambridge (198); Humphry, Mr, Cambridge (19); Hunt, Dr, Bolton (2); Hutchinson, F., London (1); Ilott, J., Whitechapel Infirmary (3); Jackson, E., London (1); James, J., London (1); Jennings, C., Tynemouth (1); Jenyns, C., Wye (1); Jeston, T., Henley (1); Johns, W. S., March (4); Johnson, G., Norwood (1); Johnston, Dr, Bradford (1); Johnstone, A., Brighton (1); Jones, J., Glamorgan (1); Jones, J., Cardiff (1); Jordison, C., Malpas (1); Kaufmann, O., Manchester (1); Kenny, Dr, Dublin (2); Kinder, R., Haddenham (3); Lancaster, Dr, London (1); Legard, W., Kirkby Lonsdale (1); Lidwell, T., Morecambe (1); Lloyd, Dr, Lambeth (7); Lloyd, T., Market Drayton (2); Longstaff, Dr, Warnswater (1); Lovegrove, Dr, Wales (1); Lucas, Mr, Huntingdon (2); Lunn, J., London (3); Lynch, Dr, London (1); Lynch, J., Sudbury (2); Maccormac, Dr, Belfast (1); Macdonald, Mr, Penrith (1); Macdonald, Dr, Dorset Asylum (2); Mackenzie, Dr, Glossop (1); Mackenzie, Dr, Rugby (4); Maclagan, Dr, Riding Mill (1); Macnicol, H., Dalmalley (1); Maguire, T., Stony Stratford (2); Manby, A., Reedham (4); Marten, P., Abingdon (1); Marten, R., Cambridge (1); Martin, J., Portlaw (2); Mathews, Dr, Redditch (1); Maude, A., Barnsley (2); Maunsell, Dr, Welford (2); May, Dr, Maldon (1); Mickley, Dr, St Luke's (4); Moore, Thomas, Blackheath (2); Molony, J., Collooney (3); Morgan, J., Langford (2); Muriel, C., Norwich (1); Newman, Dr, Stamford (3); Nicolls, W., Cork (9); Oldman, C., Bletchingley (1); Ogden, C., Rochdale (1); Palmer, J., London (1); Parry, R., Lydbury (1); Parsons, Dr, Dover (8); Pearse, Dr, Hazlemere (2); Pearson, Dr, London (1); Peart, Dr, North Shields (2); Penny, Dr, London (1); Philpot, Benjamin, Surbiton (1); Pike, Dr, Malvern (1); Plowright, C., Lynn (4); Plummit, W. G., London (3); Power, H., London (4); Rands, St J., Ipswich (4); Ransome, Dr, Bowdon (12); Reardon, D., London (1); Redwood, Dr, Rhymney (4); Reeve, Dr, Chelsea (1); Reid, Dr, Wales (1); Renshaw, Mr, Buckhurst (4); Rice, L. A., Steventon (2); Rich, Dr, Liverpool (3); Robey, Mr, Basford (1); Robinson, Dr, London (2); Rolleston, Dr, Cambridge (1); Ronaldson, J., Haddington (3); Rope, H., Shrewsbury (3); Ross, Dr, Brighton (4); Ryder, G., Sale (1); Salter, J., Basingstoke (1); Sanders, Dr, Bethnal Green (10); Sanders, Dr, London (1); Shean, Dr, Cardiff (2); Siddely, T., Bowdon (1); Sinclair, G., Kirkwall (1); Smalley, H., Dover (1); Smith, H., Notting Hill, London (1); Smith, Dr, Pershore (2); Smith, Dr, Newport, Essex (1); Stear, H., Saffron Waldon (4); Steer, A., Jamaica (1); Stevens, E., Doddington (11); Street, Dr, Oxford (1); Stretton, S., Kidderminster (1); Strover, H., Girtford (2); Sturton, Dr, Norwood (1); Sutton, J., London (1); Thomas, T., Rhymney (1); Thomson, W., Ampthill (2); Tidswell, T., Morecambe (1); Turner, Dr, Hoddes-

don (4); Tyacke, Dr, Chichester (6); Tyson, W., Folkestone (1); Vincent,
H., East Dereham (2); Vinery, Mr, Chertsey (1); Vores, Dr, Yarmouth (1);
Voss, H., Reading (1); Walford, Dr, London (2); Walker, Dr, Peter-
borough (1); Walker, Dr, Wooler (1); Ward, Dr, Oxford (1); Ward, Dr,
Leeds (1); Warren, W., Grosmont (4); Watson, Dr, Sunderland (3);
Weale, A., London (1); Weaver, Dr, Frodsham (1); Webster, Dr, London
(2); Wells, Dr, Beckshill (3); Whipham, Dr, London (1); Whittle, Dr,
Liverpool (1); Whitty, Dr, Hunstanton (1); Wilks, Dr, Ashford (13);
Williams, Dr, Wheatley (1); Williams, W. G., Wales (5); Williams, C.,
Norwich (1); Williams, O., Holyhead (12); Williamson, Dr, Ventnor (3);
Wilson, E., Cheltenham (2); Wilson, Dr, Wolverhampton (1); Wilson,
J., Liverpool (1); Woodd, H., Calstock (1); Woosman, Mr, Brecon (1);
Worthington, James, Lowestoft (3).

CONTENTS.

CHAPTER IX.

ILLUSTRATIONS.

CHAPTER I.

OLD AGE.

(THE ANNUAL ORATION DELIVERED BEFORE THE MEDICAL
SOCIETY OF LONDON, ON MONDAY, MAY 4, 1885.)

*Senile development, or decline; it, as well as disease, little, if at all,
witnessed in the struggle-for-existence-realm of nature, but carried
out under the protective influences of civilisation. Requisites for
longevity. Longevity greater in women than in men. Senile
changes, in the skeleton, the thigh-bone, the skull, the cartilages,
the arteries, the pulse, the breathing, the brain, and the bladder.
Reparative power, after wounds, fractures, and illnesses.*

OLD age acquires a gradually increasing interest, as advancing civilisation enables a larger number of persons to
attain to it, and affords them additional means of enjoying
it and profiting by it. From the schoolboy-day, now full
fifty years ago, when the *De Senectute* of the great Roman
orator made a lasting impression upon me, the subject
of old age has had some fascination for me, though multi-
farious avocations have prevented my giving much attention to it. In the past year, the Collective Investigation
Committee of the British Medical Association, at my
instance, commenced an inquiry respecting aged persons,

H. C.   1

and issued a form, with a memorandum, for the purpose of collecting information of various kinds respecting the condition, habits, etc., past and present, of persons who had attained to advanced age. The minimum age for the subjects of inquiry was fixed at 80. We are indebted to many members of the profession, and to some others, for the returns they have taken the trouble to make, which at the present exceed 500[1], the number of males and of females being nearly equal. These have been, in part, carefully tabulated and analysed by myself, with the aid of my friend and assistant, Mr A. Francis. It is not to be supposed that from this, or other investigations of the like kind, any very startling results will be obtained; for the hill of knowledge is mounted with slow and laborious steps; and we must be content to advance little by little. Moreover, I do not propose to weary you with many of the details of this inquiry, which, I may observe, is not yet completed, but to make a few remarks upon the subject of old age, which will be to some extent based upon information derived from the inquiry just mentioned.

We are, I think, too much accustomed in our ideas to limit the work of development to the periods of adolescence and maturity; and, indeed, the surpassing wonders of that work — I say surpassing wonders, for,

---

[1] They are now nearly 900.

unquestionably, the processes of development of an animal body are the most marvellous, the most mysterious, and the most interesting in the whole range of the physical world—are most fully demonstrated in the early periods of life. But they do not end in them, nor even when the body has been brought to its fully matured condition. They continue in a definite and orderly manner, though with lessened and lessening activity, to the termination of life, at whatever period that termination may, occur. The march of changing events in the human body, from the age of 40 or 50 to 100, is as regular, as orderly, as developmental, though less quick, and therefore less apparent, as it is from birth to adolescence, or from conception to birth. It is one of the resultants of that inscrutable *vis*, call it what you will, and refer it to what you will, which makes all nature one, which determines the course and end of each animate and inanimate object and by which, in the well-known words of Keble,

"To its funeral pile this aged world is borne."

A main feature of the "ascending," if we may so call it, development—the development from birth to maturity —is an increase of material, an increase of activity, and an increase of strength—of passive or resisting, as well as of active, strength; and the main feature of the "descending" development—the development from maturity

1—2

onwards—is a lessening of material, a lessening of activity, and a lessening of strength. In the normal "ascending" development, material and strength are added to the several parts of the body in due relation to their respective requirements, so that they may all grow on *pari passu*, and the proper harmony of proportion may be maintained between them ; and in the normal "descending" development, the relative proportions of the several structures and organs are preserved, while weight, force, and activity are being lowered by gradual and well-adjusted diminution of material and of nutritive activity. During the time that the bones are becoming lighter and less capable of offering resistance, the muscles become, in like proportion, lighter and weaker, and with a narrowing range of action ; and the associated volitional and other nerve-apparatus exhibits a corresponding lowering of energy and force. The loss of will to run, jump, and indulge in athletic sports is, or should be, commensurate with the inability of the muscles to effect the requisite movements, and of the bones to bear the requisite shocks. There should not even be a sigh for what is gone, or a longing for its return, though great—perhaps greater than ever— may be the pleasure in beholding the perfection of bodily form, and in witnessing the manifestations of strength and activity in the supple frames of the young. The weakening of the heart and the diminished elasticity of the arteries provide a proportionately feebler blood-current; and a lower digestive power and a lessened appetite provide a smaller supply of fuel to feed, not enough to choke, the slowing fires. Thus the capacity for action is diminishing, and the demand for it and the material for it are diminishing also; and all are diminishing in due ratio to one another. It may be said, indeed, that at all periods of life the healthy and well-working, and especially the enduring, quality of the body, depends upon a good adjustment, a good balance, of the several parts; and it is upon the well-ordered, proportionately or developmentally regulated, decline in the several organs, that the stages which succeed to maturity are safely passed, and that crown of physical glory—a healthy old age—is attained.

A time comes at length when, in the course of the descending developmental processes, the several components of the machine, slowly and much, though equally, weakened, fail to answer to one another's call, which is also weakened, a time when the nervous, the circulatory, and the respiratory organs have not force enough to keep one another going; then the wheels stop rather than are stopped, and a developmental or physiological death terminates the developmental or physiological decay. The old man who had gone to bed, apparently much as usual, is found dead in the morning, as though life's engine had been unable to repair itself in sleep suffici-

ently to bear the withdrawal of the stimulus of wake-
fulness. Or some exertion may be followed by too great
exhaustion. Dr Willis, the attendant upon King George
III., at the age of 90, after a walk of four miles to see
a friend, sat down in his chair and went to sleep, or was
thought to be asleep, but he did not wake again. Or
some slight, unusual, scarcely noticed excitement may
have the same result. A cattle-dealer, aged 98, who
attended Norwich Cattle Market on a Saturday in
December of last year, soon after talking and laughing
somewhat heartily with a few friends on the following
Tuesday, was found to be dead. Or, a slight indisposition, further lowering the status and force of some organ,
fatally disturbs the feebly maintained equilibrium. A
lady, aged 94, attended the early service at church,
walking a distance of a quarter of a mile, to and fro,
caught a slight cold, and died in the night.

How much may those who pass gently into this
natural or physiological death, be envied by the many
sufferers under the protracted and painful pathological
processes which too often induce a premature extinction
of life! The most distressing part of medical duty is the
being called upon to witness, with the inability to arrest,
the onward course of disease, such, for instance, as that
of a slowly but surely growing cancer, boring its way into
the strong and sturdily resisting frame; and the great

hope and aim of medical study is to prevent such fatal interferences with the developmental processes, and to enable these processes to work out, in their own uninterrupted way, the quiet, easy, gradual method of dissolution.

Yet, strange and paradoxical as it may seem, this gradual natural decay and death, with the physiological processes which bring them about, do not appear to present themselves in the ordinary economy of Nature, but to be dependent upon the sheltering influences of civilisation for the opportunity to manifest themselves, and to continue their work. For the needs of the first, or infantile, period of animal helplessness, Nature has made a sufficient provision in the parental instinct which protects and nurtures the young. But this lasts only so long as the requirement for it exists. It ceases as soon as the young animal has the ability to help itself; and it does not return, and is not supplemented by anything of its kind. It gives way before that struggle for existence which is the engenderer of selfishness, which dominates over all other impulses and shuts out all heed for the worn and weary, for the feeble and the decaying. These, being unable to help themselves, are crushed out by the various provisions which Nature makes for their destruction. The good result of this great seeming evil is that all in the natural, or primitive, animal world is in the ascendant to, or in the enjoyment of, bodily perfection.

All teems with budding life, or full health and strength. To falter is to fall; forasmuch as the first evidences of weakness and the beginning of decay arrest themselves by preventing the power of self-maintenance in the weak and the decaying.

The same with disease. It, in like manner, stops itself. Indeed, it scarcely can be said to be allowed to enter into the pure realm of Nature. Sick animals are not there provided for, have no abiding place there, and soon perish; so that there is no wasting and pining, no lingering fevers, no destroying cancers, no decrepid frames. Neither the bird that fails to elude the ˙hawk, nor the hawk that fails to seize the bird, can long continue in existence. Each animal has its so-called enemy ready and at watch to deliver it from feebleness and disease; and the sudden destruction which awaits them all, without fearful premonition, and with little pain— this killing in lieu of death—instead of being, as it is sometimes regarded, a cruel feature in Nature's plan, is a happy provision for deliverance from the slower death which increasing failure or progressing disease would have involved, and which civilisation entails.

Thus, in the economy of Nature, death is swift, and comes early, as soon, at least, as failure of strength renders the animal unable to protect, or provide for, itself; and man, it would seem probable, had originally

no exemption from this sharp, though, on the whole,
beneficent law of animal life. In early times, when the
race was to the physically strongest, when health, and
strength, and activity were necessary to provide the
hand-to-mouth means of sustenance and to give defence,
when men and animals were much on a par in this and
many other respects, early death must have been the
common fate, being brought about by climacteric
agencies, or by the tooth of the hungry beast, or by the
hand of man himself. This, indeed, we still find to be
the case among some of the rude races of mankind.
But in man was the germ of a better order of things,
the germ of sympathy with, of feeling and love for,
others, which was beside and above the mere parental
instinct, and which was calculated to counteract and
over-ride the selfish bent and to raise man in this, as
in some other respects, above the mere animal. This
has already done much, and it has still an ample field
for future development. Through the growth of this
germ it was given to man to introduce a new factor into
the economy of Nature, and, by forethought, by mutual
co-operation, and by care for others, which are the very
essence, at any rate the very best feature, of civilisation,
to prolong life, when, by this forethought and sympathy,
life had become more valuable, and when the prolongation of it had, consequently, become more desirable; and

scope was thus afforded for the carrying out of those descending or senile developmental processes which must have been nearly dormant in the earlier periods of human existence.

It was not to be expected that this good seed should be without a blending with tares; and the scope thus given for the fuller development of the physiological processes gave scope also for the development of the pathological processes, and enabled the various diseases to spring up and take their course, afflicting not man only, but those animals also which come under his fostering or protecting influence.

It may therefore be said that the prolongation of life into and through the periods of decay, and into and through the processes of disease—indeed almost, if not quite, the very existence of decay and disease—are the result of human forethought and sympathy. In other words, decay and disease are, by civilisation, substituted for quick and early death. Without attempting to balance the pros and cons of this, we know it to be a position from which there is not, and ought not to be, any disposition to recede; and if there were the wish, there is not the possibility. The onward march of civilisation is a necessity, and the onward progress of disease will tend to go with it. But it does remain for forethought and sympathy to narrow the range of the evils

they have themselves engendered, or which have sprung
up with them; and it is pre-eminently the noble work
of our profession to contribute to this—to weed out, and
check the growth of, the morbid tares, and to help the
good seed to grow on to its full harvest—to prevent, that
is, the origin, and to arrest the advance, of disease, and
to give to the body the best opportunities for health and
longevity. In this great physical work, let it be remembered, we shall not, to any great extent, succeed, unless
our efforts be accompanied by equal efforts to carry out
the higher and more important work of removing those
impurities in the moral atmosphere, for which civilisation has much to answer, and with which the sources
and spread of disease are closely—more closely, perhaps,
than we think—associated.

The first requisite for longevity must clearly be an
inherent or inborn quality of endurance, of steady persistent nutritive force, which includes reparative force and
resistance to disturbing agencies, and a good proportion
or balance between the several organs. Each organ must
be sound in itself, and its strength must have a due
relation to the strength of the other organs. If the heart
and the digestive system be disproportionately strong,
they will overload and oppress the other organs, one of
which will soon give way; and, as the strength of the
human body, like that of a chain, is to be measured by

its weakest link, one disproportionately feeble organ en-
dangers or destroys the whole. The second requisite is
freedom from exposure to the various casualties, indiscretions, and other causes of disease to which illness and
early death are so much due. Now, in both these—
notably in the second—woman has the advantage over
man, and she consequently attains to greater age. In
the report of the Registrar-General for 1873, eighty-nine
persons were returned as dying at or over the age of
100. Of these, ten only were males; and the superiority
of female life is well known by insurance-offices to exist,
notwithstanding the higher rate of mortality thåt has
been observed during the child-bearing period, and which,
there is good reason to think, is now, under improved
treatment, much diminishing. That this superiority is
not entirely due to the comparative freedom from exposures and to the greater temperance in the woman,
but is partly a result of a stronger or more enduring
inherent vitality, is shown by the fact that, even in the
first year of life, when the conditions and exposures of
male and female infants are the same, the mortality of
girls is less than that of boys. A somewhat larger
number of boys are born, but they are more difficult to
rear; so that the females soon gain the numerical lead,
and maintain it, with almost steadily increasing ratio, to
the end. The greater mortality of male infants in com-

parison with the female may be to some extent attributable to the larger size of the head in the former and
the consequent greater and more prolonged pressure
which it undergoes during birth. This, however, would
apply chiefly to the mortality occurring soon after birth.

This superiority may be to some extent associated
with the less wear and tear in the smaller machinery of
the woman's frame as compared with that of man; and
one might expect that the small persons in both sexes
would live longer than those of greater stature. This,
however, scarcely seems to be the case. We find from
our returns that the average height of the woman above
80 is about 5 ft. 3 in., which, allowing an inch or more
for the shortening incidental to age, makes it to fall
little, if at all, under the average middle-age stature.
The men also we find to be 5 ft. 6 in., which, making a
corresponding allowance, gives them a good average
height. It may also be observed, which we should not
have expected, that the rate both of the pulse and of
the respiration is quicker in the longer-lived sex. The
average pulse in the woman over 80 is 78 to 79, while
that in the men is 73; and the respiration in women is
22, while that in the men is 18 to 19.

It is a point of interest, in connection with the inborn, or hereditary, quality, that phthisis is reported to
have appeared in some of the immediate relatives—

father, mother, brothers, or sisters—of 82 of the 500
aged persons, namely, in 51 of the relations of the females, and in 31 of those of the males. In the reports
of some of these, it is stated to have occurred in several
members of the family; and, in a few instances, the
disease was manifested in both father and mother.   It
is evident, therefore, that the delicacy, or peculiarity,
whatever it be, of constitution, which is associated with
the tendency to the development of tubercle, is not only
not incompatible with longevity, but is not unfrequently
associated with it.

No other special peculiarities have been shown in
sufficient numbers to deserve notice here.   The greater
proportion are reported to be of long-lived families, to
have enjoyed good health throughout their lives, to have
had good appetite and good digestion, requiring little or
no medicine, to have been moderate or small eaters, to
have taken little alcohol, and, commonly, not much meat;
they have been good sleepers; and they show no traces
of gouty or rheumatic affection in the joints of the hands,
which may be taken as a fair measure of the tendency
to the disease in the various parts of the body.

I have said that the main features in the downward,
or senile, developmental process are a diminution of
material, and a diminution of force; and I apprehend
that, in the normal state, it should be simply this—such

a diminution, with, perhaps, a slight addition to the amount of oily matter naturally existing in the tissues; and that the other changes and degenerations that are incidental to age are no part of, but are rather to be regarded as deviations from, or morbid departures from, the natural phenomena.

Let us consider the changes which take place in the skeleton, forasmuch as they are the most appreciable, and, in many respects, the most interesting. The bones which, up to maturity, had been gaining in weight and size, now gradually lose weight, but do not ordinarily diminish in size; indeed, they not unfrequently rather increase in size, from the continuance of a slow process of subperiosteal ossification. To this, in part, may be attributed the sharp outlines which the figure of old persons commonly acquires, except in the case of those who become corpulent. The absorption takes place first and chiefly in the interior of the bones and in the more vascular and cancellous parts of the interior, the bony plates in these parts becoming thinned and removed, and the spaces and the canals being enlarged and filled with marrow, while the bony tissue itself becomes often, though not always, more impregnated with oily matter. Hence, although the walls of the shaft, throughout the whole length of the bones, are being gradually thinned from within, the ends of the bones, which are to a large extent cancellous, are first and most affected; and this explains the greater liability to fractures near the joints in old persons than in the middle-aged. This change, with the proportionate liability to fracture, is especially remarkable in the trochanteric part and neck of the thigh-bone, the strength of which is so much dependent upon the strength and disposition of the cancellous plates. (See photographs with description at the end of the book.)

This change takes place earlier in women than in men, which may be a consequence of the earlier cessation of active occupation in them, and the less amount of outdoor exercise they usually take; or it may be due to some natural predisposition in them, associated with a greater tendency to adipose degeneration in other parts, and evincing itself, occasionally, in an exaggerated manner, in the production of osteomalacia. The greater frequency of fracture of the neck of the thigh-bone in them is then to be attributed to the greater weakening which the part thus undergoes, as well as to the more near approach to a right angle which the neck naturally forms with the shaft in women than in men.

The vascular and cancellous character of the alveolary processes of the maxillary bones renders these parts peculiarly liable to undergo wasting or absorption, causing the loosening and falling out of the teeth, so that they commonly come out whole, or with only slight absorption of the fangs. This takes place earlier in women than in men. The average number of teeth, according to our returns, in men above 80, is 6, and in women, 3. Of 221 males, 57 are reported to be edentulous, and of 234 females, 113 are said to be in that condition. The processes of absorption and loosening of the teeth also bear a relation to the sponginess of the alveolary processes, being greatest in the upper jaw, in which the teeth, in 455 of our octogenarians, respecting whom an account of the teeth is given, are 736, those in the lower jaw amounting to 975. For the same reason, they are greater in the molar and premolar regions than in the incisor and canine, the numbers of teeth remaining being 559 molars and premolars, 409 canine, and 743 incisors.

This absorption of the alveolary processes, and consequent removal of a part of the bodily machine which is in full and daily use, is remarkable, though it has something of a parallel in the removal of another cuticular appendage; namely, the hair of the head. For the reasons I have given, it can scarcely take place in the condition of struggle for existence of the natural animal world, or in man in his primitive state; and it is, accordingly, commonly observed that the unearthed skulls of our early ancestors are well provided with teeth. The loss of teeth would imply a decay which the early man could scarcely have survived. What effect, in more modern life, this loss has upon the general health and the duration of the body, is not easy to determine. It is often survived for many years; and it may be noted that, as before stated, it takes place more in women than in men, though they are the longer-lived. Civilisation is doing something to supply the deficiency which it thus brings in its train, by providing artificial substitutes which are, at any rate, free from some of the disadvantages, such as disease and decay, associated with the natural organs.

It is remarkable how completely the alveolary processes become cleared away, so that scarcely a trace of them remains above or below. The whole framework of the face, which ministered with them to mastication, is attenuated, and the body of the lower jaw is reduced to the narrow bar of its hard lower margin. At the same time, the resistance of the teeth being removed, the direction of the pull of the muscles upon the jaw is altered, so as to open out the angle of the bone and bring its ramus and its body almost into a horizontal line. Thus the form of the lower jaw returns nearly to that of the infant. But there is this great difference; that, whereas in the infant, the bone consists mainly of the tooth-bearing, or alveolary part, and the subalveolary portion scarcely exists; in the senile condition the latter only remains, the former having been cleared away. (See Plate with description at the end of the book.)

A similar alteration of form in a bone, due to an alteration in the direction of muscular force, or to pressure from other cause, may, as we know, be produced in any part of the skeleton, and at any time of life; and, a very analogous change to this in the lower jaw may be observed to take place in the neck of a thigh-bone after amputation in the thigh; for, the nearly horizontal pull of the muscles upon the trochanter, not being resisted by the vertical weight of the body upon the head and shaft of the bone will have the effect of widening, or opening out the angle. Some years ago I placed, in the pathological museum at Cambridge, two specimens illustrating this; and the fact is not without its interest in connection with the often debated question, whether the converse of this change takes place in old age, that is, whether the angle between the neck and the shaft of the thigh-bone becomes lessened. A change of the kind certainly takes place in the ascending period of life, the angle being widest in infancy and lessening during growth; and this change is more marked in females than in males, the difference in the angle of the thigh-bone between the two sexes taking place, in all probability, about the time of puberty, when the pelvis is widening in the female, and the hips are becoming more prominent. But, does this alteration continue in the descending period? I have taken some pains to ascertain this, and have made several

2—2

measurements of the angle at the junction of the neck
with the shaft of the thigh-bone in old people; and
though I have, in some instances, found it less than in
the adult, in the greater number of cases it was not so.
I have not had the opportunity of making sufficient
measurements to settle the question; but, so far as my
observation goes, the change is the exception rather than
the rule; and I am not aware that a change of the kind
takes place in any other bone as a mere consequence of
senility, without, that is to say, there being some alteration in the direction of the pressure or forces exerted upon
the bone[1]. In the bent back of old age, the vertebræ
become modified in form; but this is a consequence of
the stoop, from enfeebled action of the dorsal muscles,
throwing the weight of the trunk too much upon the
fore part of the spinal column.

The changes which take place in the skull, during
old age, are interesting. Commonly they correspond with
those in the facial part, and the whole cranium becomes
lighter and thinner, and, therefore, smaller. In some
cases, however, it acquires an increase of thickness, by
deposit of bone on the interior of the brain-case, and
chiefly of the calvarial dome, or part, which seems to
depend upon the lessened pressure there, and the con-

---

[1] See further observations since made on this in *Journal of Anatomy
and Physiology* xxiii. 273.

sequently greater afflux of blood, caused by the shrinking
of the brain. The increase is usually most marked in the
frontal region, which accords with the fact that the
shrinking is most pronounced in the frontal lobes of
the brain. In not a few instances I have found, as
mentioned in my *Treatise on the Skeleton,* that there has
also been an increase in the density and weight of the
brain-case to such an extent that, in spite of the loss of
the teeth and of the alveolary processes of the jaws, and
the atrophy of the face, the weight of the entire skull
exceeded that of the average adult skull. In a woman, reputed to be 103, the contrast between the thick,
dense, heavy skull, and the extremely attenuated light
thigh-bone (see photograph), both of which are in the
Cambridge Museum of Anatomy, is very striking. In
connection with this change and the cause to which it
is referred, it may be observed that other parts of the
osseous system, particularly the harder parts, are liable
to undergo similar changes, leading to enlarged and
sclerotic conditions, when, at any period of life and
from any cause, they are subject to an increase of blood-
supply.

The cartilaginous parts of the skeleton become somewhat thinner, which partly accounts for the loss of height
in the aged ; but I do not think that they usually undergo any other perceptible change in ordinary healthy old

age. I have invariably found the costal cartilages soft
in old people in whom I have had an opportunity of
making an examination after death; the body of Old
Parr, as described by Harvey, therefore presenting in
this respect, as I believe, no exception to the general
rule. And I regard the calcification of them to be
a morbid rather than a senile change—a degenerative
change to which the body is liable, as it is to cataract,
bronchitis, and some other conditions, when it has passed
maturity; and not one of the natural senile developmental processes. At whatever period of life it occurs—
and it is not unfrequent about 60—it omens ill for the
further prolonged wear of the fabric. It is not quite
easy to put the condition of these cartilages to the test,
especially in elderly persons. It may, perhaps, be best
done by estimating the elasticity perceived when gentle
pressure is made upon the lower part of the sternum,
though there are obvious difficulties and objections to
this method; and, of 274 returns in our inquiry upon
this point, it is as much as can be expected that the
elasticity should be stated to be distinct in 126; in the
remaining 148, it is said to be indistinct.

It may, I think, in like manner, be said, with regard
to the calcification of the arteries, that it is the result
of a morbid process intruding itself upon, interfering with,
and arresting, the normal progress of senile development.

That it is not, at any rate to a perceptible amount, a usual accompaniment of old age, is shown by the fact that, in 362 returns respecting the condition of the arteries in persons over 80, these vessels are stated to be knotty in only 40, and to be even in 257; they are noted as being tortuous in 71. Moreover, the pulse is reported as compressible in 311, and incompressible in 72, in the returns relating to it. In the great majority of cases, therefore, the arterial system appears to present a healthy condition in those who attain to great age.

The rate of the heart's beats, according to our returns, does not vary much as age advances. From 80 to 90, it averages 73 to 74 in men, and 78 to 79 in women. It is stated to be regular in 322, and irregular or intermitting in 85.

The respiration in 110 returns of men between 80 and 85 averages 17 per minute. In 47 returns of men between 85 and 90, it averages 19 to 20; and in 16 returns of men at and over 90, it averages 23; in women, it is a little quicker. Thus, in 86 returns of women between 80 and 85, it averages 22; in 54 between 85 and 90, it is also 22; and in 37 at and over 90, it is 23. It has to be borne in mind, however, that the not unfrequent occurrence of bronchitis in the aged raises somewhat the average rate of respiration in them.

The failure of nutritive force in the brain manifests

itself in the lessening of that power of concentration and
quickness of attention upon which the sharp stamping of
impressions and the ready recall of them depend; hence
the memory for recent events is commonly impaired.
The old man meanders on in his conversation, unconscious
that he is repeating himself; he remembers the tales of
long past times, but forgets that he has just told them.
This may go on to the condition of senile dementia.
Happily, it does not often do so; and it is satisfactory
to note how many of the very aged are in good possession
of their mental faculties, taking a keen interest in passing
events, forming a clear judgment upon them, and full of
thought for the present and future welfare of others. It
is no less satisfactory to find that the active, even severe
and long-continued, functional activity of the matured
brain seems in no way to impair its enduring qualities,
and that good, earnest, useful employment of body and
mind are not only compatible with, but even conducive
to, longevity. A good example of this preservation of
mental and bodily faculty to extreme old age was presented by Titian, who is related to have been engaged
in painting a picture (his "Pieta"), which has its place
in the gallery at Venice, when, in his ninety-ninth year,
he was cut off by the plague; and this picture is said
to "tell still of incomparable steadiness of hand." The
wasting of the cerebral hemispheres, which is the accom-

paniment of failure and feebleness of the intellectual
powers, diminishes the pressure in the cranial cavity, and
so causes an increase of fluid in the subarachnoid lymph-
spaces between the convolutions, and sometimes, as I have
already mentioned, an increase in the thickness of the
skull. A similar effusion into the connective tissue of
other parts of the body, especially the lower limbs, probably, also, from deficiency of pressure upon the vessels,
or lowered tension of the several tissues, is liable to take
place, constituting a "senile œdema." This is no uncommon thing in the aged, and is sometimes induced by
temporary causes, so that recoveries from it are not unfrequent.

Of the 157 males from 80 to 85, only six are stated to
have, or to have had, disease of the prostate or bladder;
and, of these, three had recovered from it, one at the age
of 79, although the trouble had been of six years' duration.
In one, the difficulty of micturition had existed for thirty
years. Thus far, the evidence was favourable, and gave
rise to a hope that, when a certain period of life had
been attained, this serious and painful malady would be
escaped. I find, however, that of the 72 males between
85 and 90, 17 are reported to be more or less sufferers
from urinary troubles. In four of these, micturition is
stated simply to be slow. In others, there is more or less
irritability, or incontinence, or retention. One gentleman

of 88 has been entirely dependent upon the catheter for forty years. In one only of the 30 returns of men above 90 is there any mention of affection of this kind. On the whole, therefore, although the prospect of escape from diseases of the bladder and prostate gland is not quite as good as I had anticipated from the returns of the men between 80 and 85, it is evident that the aged are, to a considerable extent, free from this source of trouble. Indeed, the aged body does not seem to be, on the whole, prone to disease. Few of the returns indicate the presence of any special malady. We know that even cancers, when they attack old persons, often make slow progress in them, and sometimes fail to make way at all, remaining stationary, or even withering; and the susceptibility to contagious diseases appears to decrease from infancy to old age. The nutritive processes seem to be most easily led astray in early life, when they are in greatest activity, when there is most receptivity and excitability, and most quick communication of impressions from part to part, and from organ to organ.

In the *British Medical Journal* of the 12th July 1884, I offered some remarks on the repair of wounds and fractures in aged persons. I had frequently noticed that it, as well as the healing of ulcers, takes place as quickly as in middle-life—indeed, sometimes more quickly; and I gave the results of a collective investi-

gation on a small scale, which were confirmatory of that
view. Since then, many instances have been communicated to me by medical men which lead to the same
conclusion.

I there remarked that "the statement must be qualified in a manner which savours rather of the paradoxical;
namely, that wounds in old people heal quickly, provided
they do not slough. That is to say, the apparently opposite tendencies exist at this time of life—namely, the
tendency to slough and the tendency to heal quickly.
Such, for instance, is the experience of oculists, whose
testimony on the subject I have asked. They find that
the cornea sometimes sloughs after the operation for
cataract in old people; but that, when it does not slough,
the wound heals quite as quickly as, or more quickly than,
at an earlier time of life. So in other operations. The
old person may sink, or the wound may slough or ulcerate;
but, if these eventualities be escaped, a quick healing may
be expected.

"Certainly this would not have been anticipated. We
should not have thought, when the nutritive forces are
generally failing, when strength and weight are diminishing, when repair is each year less and less able to keep
pace with wear, as evinced, among other things, by the
fact that exhaustion is more quickly induced and less
quickly recovered from; when the brain is shrinking, and

memory and other mental powers are lowering, and when
the circulation is becoming weaker—that, under these
circumstances, the nutritive or reparative processes concerned in breach-closing—in the healing of wounds and
ulcers—should manifest an increase of energy, at any
rate, of rapidity, in carrying on their work. I do not
know well how to explain it; but this exceptional phe-
nomenon of nutrition is not peculiar to old age. It
may be observed in some other lowered conditions. The
wounds in patients exhausted by large losses of blood
usually heal quickly, as they also do after operations for
cancer, and in many other debilitated conditions. I do
not mean in persons of naturally strumous temperament,
but persons who have been weakened by illness or in
other ways. So do, commonly, the gaps caused by car-
buncles, and bed-sores; and very remarkable is the quick
healing of the stump left by senile gangrene; that is to
say, this evidence of vital energy is manifested in the
part next above that which was unable to keep alive at
all. An exception must be made of certain impaired conditions of the nervous system, in which wounds and sores
are sometimes very troublesome."

The fact that the fracture of the neck of the thigh-
bone, which may be regarded as the old person's fracture,
rarely unites, will be urged in support of the opposite and
more generally accepted view on this point. "It is well

known, however," to quote again from the same paper, "that this failure depends, not upon the age of the patient, or upon any peculiarity in the structure of the bone, or upon any changes that take place in it during the later periods of life, though those changes are such as to cause rarefaction of its cancelli and greater liability to fracture, but upon other causes. Such causes, more particularly, are the separation of the broken surfaces, which commonly occurs; the buried position of the inner fragment in the cavity of the acetabulum, which prevents any overlapping of the fragments and any throwing out of uniting matter all around it; as well as the comparative absence, and, when the fibrous covering of the neck is torn through all round, the complete absence, of tissue in which that material can be produced; and also the bathing of the fractured surfaces by the synovial fluid. That these conditions, which are found to be more or less prejudicial to bony union of fractures into other joints, and not senility, are the real causes of failure in the case of the neck of the thigh-bone, is proved by the fact that union of bone will take place at this part of the skeleton as well as elsewhere, if the fractured surfaces be fixed in apposition either by any kind of impaction or by well adjusted appliances;" and that this will occur in the aged, there is ample evidence in our museums.

The same remark does not, I fear, apply to the repair

after exhaustion from fatigue. The old person is soon tired, and does not recover quickly. The restorative processes of sleep are not so brisk in him as in the young. I have often, however, been surprised at the quick recovery of health and strength by old persons who have been depressed by indisposition and illness; and I have attributed this rallying power to the general soundness of the system, and the good working balance of the several organs which has brought them to old age. To what extent it is, as a general rule, shared by the aged, and may be relied upon in them, I must leave to wider experience to decide.

After all, length of life is to be really estimated not by numbers of years so much as by good work done, not by the amount of time spent in the tame fruitless manner indicated by the pithy lines of Cowper:

> "For fourscore years this life Cleora led:
> At morn she rose, at night she went to bed;"

nor by endeavours solely to advance our own fortunes, or reputation, or comfort, but by persevering efforts to promote the welfare of our fellow-men.

Thus considered, how large have been the lives which many of you have spent in long laborious days and watchful nights, with little present gain or prospect of future requital, in the out-patient and *post mortem* rooms of our hospitals, by the midnight lamp, or by the bedsides of the sick in this vast metropolis, where civilisation has

worked out its best and its worst results. While wishing
you yet many years of the like usefulness and its assured
reward, I must express the feeling that it is not right
or just that, in this, the wealthiest city the world has
ever seen, and in this very wealthy land, so much of the
time and energies—the best time and energies—of many
of the younger members of our profession should be
devoted to attendance upon out-patients, and so much
time of a far larger number of the profession should be
employed in the onerous and anxious duties of the poor-
law service, with such very inadequate pecuniary remu-
neration. For the sake of all concerned, reform is needed
here.

I will only further add that there are many points in
relation to longevity which I have alluded to only briefly
or not at all; that it will be evident, from the few figures
that I have given, that we need more information; that
the forms and memoranda issued by the Collective
Investigation Committee can be obtained from the
Secretary to the Committee, at the office of the British
Medical Association, 161A, Strand; and that we shall be
obliged if any of those present, or other members of the
profession, will contribute to our store, especially by
making returns of persons who have attained or exceeded
the age of 90 years.

CHAPTER II.

CENTENARIANS.

CONCLUSIONS FROM THE REPORTS OF THE CONDITIONS, HABITS, FAMILY HISTORY, ETC. OF FIFTY-TWO[1] CENTENARIANS, GIVEN IN RETURNS MADE ON A FORM OF INQUIRY ISSUED BY THE COLLECTIVE INVESTIGATION COMMITTEE OF THE BRITISH MEDICAL ASSOCIATION. WITH REMARKS AND ANALYSIS[2].

IN the publication of this table[3] it is not meant to be implied that each of the fifty-two persons positively attained to the age of 100 years. Some no doubt did so; and in eleven (two males and nine females, one of these aged 108, and one 106) the age was confirmed by baptismal certificates or other records. Respecting others, there is necessarily more or less uncertainty; but these may reasonably be assumed to have reached nearly to that age. The name is given in each case; and the

---

[1] Subsequent additions which are given later have brought the number reported on up to seventy. Fifty-two, however, only were included in the table.

[2] The analysis of the table is given at p. 55.

[3] The table will be found in the Supplement to the *British Medical Journal*, Dec. 11, 1886, and in the *Collective Investigation Record*, III. 81.

names are also given of the informants. These were nearly all medical men who volunteered the information which they would not have done unless they believed it to be correct, and who, in many cases, were well acquainted with the persons respecting whom they gave the particulars. The well-known pride of longevity and the tendency to exaggerate and deal with the marvellous throw some suspicion over all records of this kind, and, indeed, had well-nigh caused a revulsion to misbelief in the capacity of the human body to retain vitality for so long a period as a hundred years. Abundant well-established examples of its doing so have, however, dissipated that scepticism which, I suppose, is now held by scarcely any one; and it has been calculated from the Reports of the Registrar-General that there is about one centenarian to every 127,000 people. It will be observed that none of the cases here given range among the marvellous and startling instances we sometimes read of[1]. Not one is stated to have reached 110; three are said to have been 108, and one 106.

---

[1] For notices of such (Epaminondas æt. 157, Parr æt. 152, Countess of Desmond, æt. 160, and others) as well for many interesting points in relation to longevity—in the ages of Bishops, Deans, Judges, Peers, and General officers, &c.—I may refer to the article by Dr J. Burney Yeo in the *Nineteenth Century*, March 1888. Henry Jenkins, a Yorkshireman, is said to have died in 1670 at the age of 169 having assisted, when a boy, in conveying arrows to Flodden Field at the battle which was fought 158 years previously. *Philosophical Transactions* XIX. 266.

H. C   3

Our thanks are due to the gentlemen who have been
so good as to take the trouble (often considerable) to gather
and give the information from which the table was made.
For assistance in compiling it, and for the analysis, I am
indebted to A. Francis, M.R.C.S., of King's College, in
this University.

I have a large collection of reports of persons between eighty and a hundred, which are all tabulated, and
the analyses of which, with remarks, will appear at a later
page; but the interest attaching to a record of so many
reputed centenarians will, I think, be deemed to justify
a separate statement respecting them.

Some reports of centenarians, which came in since the
table was in type and the analysis upon it was made, with
remarks, are given subsequently.

Though it must be granted even of the centenarian, as
of all others, that he soon "passeth away and is gone,"
yet happily we are not obliged to admit that his "strength
is but labour and sorrow." In many instances, on the
contrary, he has, if not a green, yet a mellow and cheerful
old age, one of happiness to himself and pleasure to others,
brightened by a vivid though calm interest in the present, and unshadowed by apprehension respecting the
future. "Pay me a visit when you next come to Leaming-
ton," were usually among the words of adieu by Miss

Hastings, at the age of 103, to her friends; "I shall like to see you, and hear how you are going on." There is a great moral in this; for while we are denizens in this World, we are bound to make to ourselves friends of it, which is best done by a cheerful happy use of it, and by enjoying it and using well the powers and privileges it gives us; and the injunction is none the less imperative and valuable when the sojourn in it has lasted for five score years and more. Moreover, in this, as in so many other instances, the influences are reciprocal; for, associated as cheerfulness and happiness are with good doing and kind feeling, they are also much dependent upon the smooth working of the several parts of a sound bodily machinery, to the healthfulness of which they in their turn not a little contribute. So long, indeed, as the body is enjoyable, and its functions go glibly and smoothly on, the tenant is commonly desirous of continuing its occupation. When it ceases to be so, when lassitude and weariness supervene, when means of communication with others are stopping, when the "*sans* everything" condition is impending, he is content to quit it; and when the tenement becomes distressing or painful, he is anxious to do so. Still, though the capacities for activity and work may be passing away, and life's "fitful fever" with them, the old person may comfort himself with the reflection that a useful mission still remains in the benign influence of

a serene and benevolent disposition, which calmly esti-
mates the things of time and sense at their true value,
and which, leniently regarding the shortcomings of others,
gives the true crown of glory to the hoary head.

It is most satisfactory to find that the exercise—even
the full exercise—of the various powers, mental and
bodily, is not merely compatible with, but is conducive
to, great age ; that, as has been well said, " the harmonious development of the many-sided aspects of man
is conducive to health and the prolongation of life," and
that there need be no fear of entering heartily and
actively, and with full interest and energy, into the
assigned work of life, physical or mental. The body is
made, not for ease and sloth, but for labour and play, for
work and enjoyment, better still for enjoyment of work.
Work, enjoyed as it should be, promotes health of body,
and, especially if stimulated by other motives than personal
ambition and gain, engenders that cheerful, placid frame
of mind which is one of the adjuncts of centenarianism.

France has lately celebrated the centenary of a philo-
sopher and a chemist, M. Chevreul, who the same night
occupied the President's box at the opera[1]; and we are

---

[1] We read in the *Times* of Sep. 1, 1888, that M. Chevreul enters his
103rd year; his health excellent, he eats and drinks heartily and sleeps
well, drives daily in a one horse chaise which he has had for forty years,
rises early, takes a plate of soup, goes to bed again and sleeps till noon,
then breakfasts off two eggs and minced meat, at four takes a bowl

told that a Chinese centenarian recently passed the examination which qualified him to enter the highest academy of the Mandarins. Delightful was the account of Lady Smith, in whom a bright, intelligent mind and a brisk healthy body had been in uninterrupted harmonious action for a hundred and three years, and who to the last took a lively interest in the world's political and other movements.

Among the fifty-two centenarians on our own list, the INTELLECT, in those of whom a report respecting it is given, is stated to have been high in 11 and low in 5 only. They enjoy also much of the pleasures of MEMORY, as many as thirty-nine out of forty-seven having good memory for past events, and twenty-six out of thirty-nine having that freshness which is indicated by good memory for recent events; one could quote a good deal of the Bible, and another could repeat a hundred psalms correctly. Several were remarkable for MENTAL AND BODILY ACTIVITY AND ENERGY during their long lives. Twenty are reported as strong, 16 of average strength, and 12 only as feeble. Many had been engaged in hard bodily toil, or mental work, and in various occupations and in different

of milk and two biscuits, lies down again for two hours, then has another plate of soup and goes to bed for the night. Sept. 4, he visited the Sanitary Exhibition at the Palace of Industry. Arm-in-arm with a friend he mounted the stairs and walked through the Exhibition. He reads scientific and literary works and is interested in the proceedings of scientific bodies and in recent discoveries.

ways had played their parts effectually on the world's
stage to the end of the long drama which they reached in
better plight than the well-known lines of the great poet
might lead us to expect. I often wish that Shakespeare
had lived to give a brighter version of his seven stages, and
to portray the old man not lean and slippered, but well
favoured and booted, keen in life's interest, and happy in
promoting the welfare and enjoyment of others. Even
in the bedridden state, of which our record gives seven
examples (four males and three females), one of whom
had been bedridden for seven years, all is not cheerless.
The quiet coziness, the even temperature, the freedom from
exposure, and the reservation to the vital organs of nerve-
energy and nutritive material, consequent on the diminished
use of the muscular system, contribute to prolong the
lives of some feeble persons who still retain the pleasures
of intellectual occupation and social intercourse, to say
nothing of the enjoyment of memory and sleep and the
gratification of the appetite ; and it is curious, though not
unfrequently to be observed, that continuance in bed ac-
tually increases both sleep and appetite. Some aged people
lie in bed in the winter; and, in the dull routine of the
workhouse, many old people drift into the bedridden state.

In our table, as usual in records of longevity, the
women preponderate over the men (36 to 16), in spite
of the dangers incidental to child-bearing and the diseases

associated with the varying demands made, at different periods, upon the organs connected with that process. This is obviously, in great measure, to be attributed to the comparative immunity of the woman from the exposures and risks to which man is subjected, as well as to her greater temperance in eating and drinking, and her greater freedom from the anxieties attendant upon the world's labour and business. Still, as I have said (p. 12), there appears also to be a greater inherent vitality in the female, as evinced by the fact that, even in the first year of life, when the conditions and exposures of male and female infants are the same, the mortality of girls is less than that of boys. It is also to be learned from the analysis of our reports that the ELASTICITY OF THE THORAX, as evinced by the condition of the costal cartilages, and its capacity for dilatation during inspiration, is better preserved in women than in men. In the matter of the ARCUS SENILIS, also, the woman has the advantage; but, in the condition of the arterial system, much difference is not shown.

Of the 36 women, 26 had been MARRIED, and 11 had large families; and it may be some consolation to young mothers and their friends to find that 8 of the 26 married before they were twenty—1 at 16 and 2 at 17. The dangers, happily diminishing, which are incidental to child-bearing, must not be forgotten; but, irrespective of

these, the process itself and the attendants thereon do
not seem to militate against longevity. Indeed, the
capacity for the full exercise of this, like that of the
other normal functions, is one of the qualities in those
who have the other requisites for attaining to great age.
One only of the married women was childless; but neither
the age at which she was married nor the duration of her
married life are given.

It might be anticipated, indeed, from the matrimonial
tendency, and the prolific quality evinced by the tables—
the average number of children born to each, whether
man or woman, being 6—that there would be, through
inheritance, a gradual increase in the centenarian breed;
and it is probable that this is the case, and that the
duration of life is, from this and other favouring causes,
gradually being extended. The life-period of the children
we have no means of determining with accuracy, the
returns being, from various causes, imperfect; but we
may safely accredit them with, at least, an average
longevity. It is, moreover, a point of some interest that
many of the centenarians were members of large families,
averaging, indeed, 7 or 8; those designated as "only
children" being limited to 2. Of the 52, 41 had been
married, and 11, of whom 10 were women, had remained
single; but we cannot from this draw any inference as
to influence of matrimony upon longevity. Possibly

something may be gleaned from the analysis of the numerous reports I have received of persons between 80 and 100.

The fact that 12 of these centenarians were "FIRST CHILDREN" does not accord with the idea entertained by some persons that first children are at a physical disadvantage. The generally prevalent custom of inheritance by the firstborn, and the Mosaic injunction (Exodus xiii. 2) "Sanctify unto me all the firstborn, whatsoever openeth the womb among the children of Israel, both of man and of beast, it is mine," are also scarcely in harmony with such a view. Nevertheless, some confirmation of the view is furnished by the feeling on this matter, founded, it may be presumed, on experience, in racing stables, which, I have been informed, is not in favour of firstlings.

In the case of one of our centenarians, the parents were first COUSINS.

The tables and the analyses of present and past condition yield nothing striking or even novel or unexpected, or in that respect interesting; but they are not therefore less valuable or important. The qualities that lead to great age are precisely those which might have been anticipated: a good family history; a well-made frame of average stature (5 feet 8, which is rather above the average, in the male, 5 feet 3 in the female); spare rather than stout, throughout life robust, with good health, little troubled with ailments or illnesses of any kind, with good digestion, regular daily action of bowels; active, capable of much exertion, with the restorative advantages of good sound sleep permitting or inducing early rising (not one is reported to have been a 'bad' sleeper, and nearly all were 'early risers'); good vocal organs; a good appetite moderately indulged, with little need of, and little consumption of, alcohol or animal food; an energetic yet placid temperament; a good intelligence; the hair holding its ground and its colour well; the organs of sight and hearing performing their functions well and long. Some retained great activity to the end. One woman 'danced and sung on her 101st birthday'; another 'received the holy communion in Church on her hundredth birthday'; a third 'walked in the hay-field and amused herself making hay on her hundredth birthday'; and a man aged 101 had 'walked at least 4 miles the day before the return was filled up.' Mrs Covill, of Settrington, whom I visited in her 101st year, was quite bright and brisk, able to walk about, and was engaged in the occupation, in which she evidently took a lively interest, of mending her stays. She evinced no desire for the speedy termination of her long life, confirming in this the general rule, whatever the age may be, that life is pleasant so long as the body is healthy (see account of her death, p. 86).

Our centenarians afford, in short, good examples

through life of the *mens sana in corpore sano*, of the consequent enjoyment of life and of the desire to continue it, an enjoyment which, in most cases, is in no degree lessened by the feeling of contentment to part with it whenever the time for that may come; and in by far the greater number there was a total absence of any evidence of RHEUMATIC OR GOUTY AFFECTION, past or present, in the JOINTS OF THE FINGERS—a condition which is not unfrequently regarded as one of the heralds of old age, and which, doubtless, like many other local maladies of which it may be taken as a sample, is often prophylactic against other more serious maladies. It seems that the frame which is destined for great age needs no such prophylactics, and engenders none of the peccant humours for which the finger-joints may find a vent. To have a vent for such humours may be good, but it is less good than to be without them. Of the eight in whom those joints were stiff or deformed, it may be observed that No. 1[1], a man, always "drunk as much as I could, and always will do;" a second and third (6 and 21), poor women, had been subject to much exposure and had a rough life, following the army in various parts of the world; of the case of the fourth (20), also a female, in whom these joints were stiff, we have no account of the habits. The fifth (29), a female, appears to have been a

---

[1] These numbers refer to the table already mentioned, p. 32.

temperate person in comfortable circumstances, in whom no particular reason for the deformity of the joints can be assigned; and the same may be said of the sixth and seventh (30 and 39), except that the latter was in the habit of partaking rather freely of animal food, and also probably of the eighth (49), though we have not much information as to her past habits. It is rather remarkable that all of these, except the first, are women; of these women, three were poor, and the others in comfortable or affluent circumstances.

The loss of TEETH presents some interesting problems. It seems to be an associate of civilisation, partly because the varied and peculiar conditions of civilised life tend to induce it, and partly because those conditions have the effect of preserving the body beyond the limits which, under natural or uncivilised conditions, appear to have been assigned to it. Not developed till the animal begins to care for itself, the teeth fade away when it ceases to be able to do so ; and, in the state of nature, life is not much prolonged beyond the period when the self-providing powers are waning. Civilisation, however, brings many external or extraneous aids and protections which carry the body on beyond what may be called the dental or natural span, and maintain it in spite of losses and changes which, to the uncivilised man, would have been fatal. Of these changes, the loss of teeth is one from the ill effects of which we obtain great immunity. Twenty-four of our centenarians had no teeth. Some had been without them many years, and the average number retained was only four or five, which, in many instances, we may conclude to have been of little value. Three women (Nos. 25, 34 and 39) are stated each to have retained a complete set. One woman (No. 6) had seventeen teeth, of which one only was in the upper jaw. Another (No. 7) had sixteen, and a man (No. 37) had twenty-four. Lady Smith is said in her 104th year to have preserved all her teeth as well as good eyesight. The artificial substitutes were used in so few instances, that we cannot from them form an estimate of the aid these appliances afford towards the prolongation of life ; but that they do contribute to the maintenance of health and the prolongation of life can scarcely be a matter of doubt. The teeth had disappeared, as we have before found to be the case (p. 17), in the upper jaw more than in the lower; but the tables do not show so much difference in this respect between the men and the women as there stated.

It is somewhat remarkable that, though as many as twenty-eight used glasses, thirty-five, including many who used glasses, are reported to have been in the enjoyment of good SIGHT. The occurrence of presbyopia does not seem to be associated with, or to be a prelude to, inconvenience or impairment of sight beyond that which may be corrected by glasses. These had been used by some for forty or fifty years; and in three it appears that the defect was spontaneously rectified, and that as they grew older they became able to dispense with glasses.

That the majority of centenarians are content, as we find them to be, with three meals in the day, and are moderate or small EATERS, partaking of little animal food and little alcohol, is in harmony with the lowered activity of the muscular and other organs, and the consequent lowered demand upon the nutritive processes and the nutritive supply. That nevertheless the rate of the pulse, averaging 70, and that of the respiration, averaging 22, are maintained, may be accounted for by the diminished elasticity of the circulatory and respiratory apparatus. The arteries become less capable of accelerating the blood-stream, and the vital capacity of the chest is much reduced, as shown by the slight difference.in the chest-girth between the state of inspiration and that of expiration (p. 58).

The SLEEP-DURATION, averaging nearly nine hours, indicates also a slowness, a feebleness, of the restorative processes. Repair is tardily and with difficulty striving to keep pace with wear. We know that it is one element in the developmental law of growth and decay, that the balance should not be quite maintained in the aged frame. Up to adolescence repair has the mastery, and the body gains in weight and strength; in middle age, repair is about equal to wear; but in later life its gradual failure, attended with diminishing weight and strength, conducts the body slowly along its normal course to dissolution. Long, good sleep, does something to put a drag on the downward course, and is a great sustainer of the aged frame. Much difference in sleep-duration is noted in the tables. In some, sleep is said to be short and indifferent, or bad, perhaps owing to peculiar disturbing causes; but in 32 out of the 44 in whom mention of it is made it is said to be good.

The MALADIES of these old people range themselves chiefly under the head of weakness, evinced by inability to put forth or maintain much effort of any kind, bodily or mental. Fatigue soon comes on; the muscular weakness proceeding in some cases to partial or complete loss of the use of the lower limbs, and to tremor of the upper limbs. The difficulty of penning a straight line resulting from this latter, being the cause of the smallness of the handwriting, often noticeable, of old people. The weakness of the brain evinces itself in impairment of memory, in slowness of apprehension, in inability to fix the thoughts long on one thing, and the tendency, therefore, to wander from one subject to another, and to travel to and fro, which may pass on to want of control, or imbecility, or even to dementia. This last, saddest state of all, was witnessed only in two of our centenarians. Indeed, the brain in many held out as well or better than other organs —which may be regarded one of the bright rays, if not the brightest, in the centenarian landscape.

The weakness, or failing, seems to have been about equal in the several great organs, showing that these organs presented to the last that good balance of enduring strength which is so essential to longevity. The lungs are, through life, the most sensitive to atmospheric changes, as well as to alterations in the conditions of the blood. Hence, bronchitic and pneumonic affections are a common source of distress, and a frequent cause of death at all periods of life; but it does not clearly appear that the very aged are more liable to them than those who are less advanced in years. .

In the majority, in our record, the action of the heart was regular, the pulse was small and compressible, and the evidences of arterial degeneration were not manifest. In some of those who were auscultated, more or less *bruit* was heard, indicating some valvular or arterial roughness; but it made no apparent impression, and the individuals were unconscious of any defect. The slowness of micturition mentioned in two men, and the incontinence in three females, as well as the frequency of micturition in three, may also be regarded as resulting from atony, rather than

from disease. Indeed, these old people had outlived the
period which is most liable to prostatic and other urinary
troubles. Other minor maladies and discomforts, of which
we may conclude that centenarians have their share, such
as the slight eczema in No. 3, and the flatulence in No. 4,
have, in many instances, probably been thought not worthy
of mention.

Though the majority had suffered little from illness at
former periods, some up to the very end of their long lives,
yet it is not unsatisfactory to find that the effects of illnesses, even when severe, do not always preclude longevity.
No. 1 had rheumatic fever when young, and rheumatism
afterwards; No. 5 had epilepsy from 17 to 70; No. 7 had
renal disease, with loss of sight, at 30, from which there
was complete recovery; No. 8 had an abscess connected
with the spine, a stiff knee from injury at 50, and
diarrhœa from 70 to 75, besides fevers and other ailments;
No. 9 had gall-stones at 60; No. 10 was ten years in an
asylum after a confinement; No. 11 had peritonitis; No.
12 had had fever at 25, also jaundice and small-pox;
No. 13 (Mrs Covill) had "bad stroke" at 60, for which
she was bled, and two less severe strokes at 70. No.
18 had renal dropsy at 82, lasting for two years; No. 23
had acute bronchitis at 95; No. 29 had paralysis at 90;
No. 31 had severe herpes zoster; No. 33 had rheumatic
fever at 70; No. 45 had severe bronchitis at 82; No. 51

had paralysis when a child; Nos. 6, 12, 17, and 47, had fever—12 and 47 badly.

The RECOVERIES FROM ILLNESS at great age, to which I have before called attention, are to be noted. We find that No. 18 recovered at 82 from renal dropsy which lasted two years, and at 98 recovered from a large slough on the thigh, caused by a bruise; No. 23 from acute bronchitis at 95, and pneumonia and erysipelas of the head at 99; No. 33 from rheumatic fever at 70; No. 45 from severe bronchitis at 82; and No. 47 from severe fever at 84. Six had suffered injury to the hip after the age of 90. One broke the neck of the thigh-bone at 90, and one at 101, the latter so far recovering as to go on crutches.

Most interesting and important of all are the LIFE-HABITS of these old people, among which, activity, out-of-door exercise, and early rising, with moderation in diet and alcohol, stand out in strong relief, and are evidently among the important factors in longevity. At the same time, we perceive that most of these habits may be regarded as the attributes of the well-wearing body, that is to say, they are the resultants of health, as well as the promoters of it. The healthy, vigorous body, can scarcely be otherwise than active, in one way or other; and few things tend to promote health and vigour more than activity—activity without excitement—an activity which is not forced beyond the measure of good and easy repair —an activity which does not wear the body out. The candle ought to burn briskly, and, as a general rule, at both ends, regarding the head or brain as one end, and the limbs or locomotory agents as the other; but it should not burn too fast; and it may be that, in some persons, an extra rate at one end is better to be compensated by a lower rate at the other. Some persons, at least, seem to find that severe and continued brain-work is incompatible with much leg-work. Into this question, however, I will not enter.

Most of them had been accustomed to much out-of-door exercise; and upon this, with the refreshing influence of open air, stress should be laid, for it must not be supposed that exercises and athletics in-doors, where they are much more exhausting, are a sufficient substitute, especially in the case of young and growing persons.

Such activity causes a brisk trade in the nutritive market; and the demand is pretty sure to be met by the supply, when food can be obtained. The moderation or spareness in diet, notable in the past habits of our centenarians, limiting the supply, prevents a wasteful overflooding of the market, and compels an economical and good employment of all that is brought there. Surplusage can do but harm. The body associates itself with a certain well-known evil agent in finding for idle food

4—2

"some mischief sure to do," although, in some individuals, a drainage for unused material may be made through the intestinal or renal or cutaneous organs, which, be it remembered, were never meant to serve that purpose, and which are likely to suffer from the strain thus put upon them. In many a more deleterious vent is found in gout, bilious attacks, etc., which, at the same time, exert a beneficial influence by causing a temporary arrest of supply, or in graver inflammatory attacks, or in the still graver malignant affections. The temperance in all things of our centenarians has, without doubt, been one great means of keeping order in their nutritive system, and preventing aberrations into morbid processes. Few more mischievous notions have found their way into common acceptance than the idea that strength is proportionate to the amount of food taken; and it is accepted and mischievous, no doubt, in a greater degree than it would otherwise be, because it rests upon the basis of truth that strength cannot be maintained without a sufficient supply of food.

The total abstainers will not fail to observe that twelve of our centenarians had been through life, or for a long period, in their ranks; that twenty took little ALCOHOL; that this was, in the case of some of them, *very* little; and that eight were moderate. There were however some exceptions. No. 1, who was a jolly person and sung a song at a Christmas feast, when 103, had led a rough life as a gamekeeper and was fond of drink; No. 18, who had been a collier, took beer rather freely; No. 8 often drank to excess on festive occasions; No. 14 was a free beer-drinker, though never drunk; and No. 35 "drank like a fish during his whole life," which probably means when he could, for it is added that "he could not usually get much[1]." It is, perhaps, scarcely less important to note that our centenarians were, for the most part, SMALL MEAT-EATERS.

The EARLY RISING during the greater part of life was in many of the instances necessitated by their occupations. Still, this habit must be regarded as an associate or sequence of the healthful activity just mentioned, and of an activity pervading the reparative work which has to be done in sleep—an activity which quickly and thoroughly refits the body for its next day's work, and gives the energy, the willingness, the desire to resume it. Sleep should come quickly, be intense while it lasts, and cease quickly and completely; quite awake or quite asleep; no hovering between the two; no need of, or desire for, a little more slumber, a little more sleep. "When one turns in bed, it is time to turn out," whether rightly or wrongly attributed to the Duke of Wellington, is a saying worthy

[1] Other examples of Centenarians who had been by no means abstainers are mentioned by Dr Yeo.

of him, and accords with the energy that contributed to make his life great as well as long.

The statement as to the time they had been in the habit of spending in bed is not very exactly to be relied on for many reasons. By one twelve hours was stated, by others five; seven or eight appears to have been the average.

While we thus gain more clear knowledge of the qualities for, and the adjuncts to, centenarianism, an examination of the table shows that there is no royal road to it. We see that it is attained under a variety of conditions, and that few persons can be said to be excluded from the prospect of it. With regard to certain of the important requisites, we cannot alter our position. No one can make his family history better than it is, or make his body to be wound up for a longer period than its normal life's span; but it is the duty of each to endeavour to make it cover that span and to go as long as its appointed time. The uncertainty as to that term, as it is one of the greatest blessings of life, so should it be one stimulus to us to ascertain and to follow the means most suited for prolonging life, especially as we find the result of this investigation to be that those are the means best calculated to turn it to good account and also to make it happy.

CHAPTER III.

ANALYSIS OF THE RETURNS RESPECTING FIFTY-TWO[1] CENTENARIANS.

PRESENT CONDITION.

AGE.—Fifty-two returns; average age, about $102\frac{1}{5}$ years. *Males.*—Sixteen returns; average age, about $102\frac{1}{4}$ years; respective ages, 108, 105, 104, 4 aged 103, 3 aged 102, 2 aged 101, $101\frac{1}{4}$, 4 aged 100.—*Females.*—Thirty-six returns; average age, about $102\frac{1}{6}$ years; respective ages, 2 aged 108, 1 aged 106, 3 aged 105, 3 aged 104, 4 aged 103, 4 aged 102, 7 aged 101, 12 aged 100.   In 11 cases, the age returned was verified by baptismal certificates or other records; of these, 2 were males, aged 101 and 100; and 9 were females, aged 108, 106, 104, 103, 102, 101, 101, $100\frac{1}{2}$, and 100.

MALE OR FEMALE.—Fifty-two returns; M. 16, F. 36.

SINGLE: MARRIED: WIDOWED.—Fifty-two returns; S. 11 (of these 10 were females), M. 5, W. 36.

AFFLUENT: COMFORTABLE: POOR.—Fifty returns; A. 3, C. 28, P. 19.

FAT: SPARE: AVERAGE.—Fifty returns; F. 9 (of these 8 were females), Sp. 23, A. 18.

FULL-BLOODED: PALE: AVERAGE.—Forty-six returns; F. 8, P. 14, A. 24.

STRONG: FEEBLE: AVERAGE.—Forty-eight returns; S. 20, F. 12, A. 16.

[1] The nineteen given in the following chapter make the entire number seventy-one.

FIGURE: ERECT OR BENT.—Fifty returns; E. 25, B. 25.

HEIGHT. *Males.* --Twelve returns; average, about 5 ft. 8½ in.; one also returned as short. *Females.*—Twenty-six returns; average about 5 ft. 3 in.

WEIGHT. *Males.*—Seven returns; average nearly 138 lbs. *Females.*—Ten returns: average about 129 lbs. Respective Weights. *Males.*—182, 165, 147, 140, 120, 112, 98 lbs. *Females.*—196, 154, 140, 136, 126, 126, 120, 112, 112, 70 lbs.

VOICE.—Forty-seven returns; loud, 6; clear, 16; weak, 7; full, 3; loud and clear, 8; full and clear, 6; loud and full, 1.

HEARING.—Forty-nine returns; good, 22; indifferent, 17; bad, 9; deaf, 1.

JOINTS.—Forty-seven returns; natural, 37; stiff, 4; deformed, 3; stiff and deformed, 1; the last was stiff from chronic rheumatism, and deformed from contraction of palmar fascia; slightly deformed, 2; one of these was 'from rheumatoid arthritis.'

SIGHT.—Fifty-one returns; of these, 34 had good sight; 6 had cataracts, in one case unilateral, in another commencing; in 8 others, failure of eyesight was reported, apparently independent of presbyopia.

GLASSES.—Thirty-five returns; 28 used glasses, 7 did not, but of these 4 were returned as 'poor,' and were possibly unable to read; 6 had used them for 40—50 years, 5 for 30—35 years, 4 for 10—20 years, 2 for 4—6 years, 5 for 'many years,' 2 for 'few years.' One had used spectacles for many years, but for the last twelve years had been able to read without them; another had not used them for twelve years; another 'not for many years,' but one 'cannot now get them strong enough.'

DIGESTION.—Forty-seven returns; good, 40; moderate, 7.

APPETITE.—Forty-eight returns; good, 36; bad, 2; moderate, 10.

EATER.—Forty-six returns; moderate, 25; small, 9; large, 12.

NUMBER OF MEALS DAILY.—Forty-three returns; average number rather more than 3 daily; the greatest number was 5 daily (in 1 case); the least number was 2 daily (in 5 cases).

ALCOHOL.—Forty-six returns; none, 15; little, 24; moderate, 6; great deal of beer, 1.

ANIMAL FOOD.—Forty-one returns; none, 3; moderate, 10; little, 25; very little, 2; much, 1.

BOWELS.—Forty-three returns; daily, 26; alternate days, 6; irregular, 11.

APERIENTS.—Forty-one returns; rarely, 22; never, 14; frequently, 5.

DISPOSITION.—Forty-six returns; placid, 14; irritable, 8; energetic, 11; placid and energetic, 8; irritable and energetic, 5.

INTELLECT.—Forty-six returns; average, 29; low, 5; high, 11; childish for 6 years, 1. One was said to be 'slow in comprehending questions, but smart in reply.'

MEMORY. Recent Events.—Thirty-nine returns; good, 26; bad, 6; moderate, 7. Past Events.—Forty-seven returns; good, 39; bad, 4; moderate, 4. One 'remembers and will quote a great deal of the Bible,' another 'could repeat about 100 Psalms correctly.'

HABITS.—Forty-eight returns; active, 26; sedentary, 15; bedridden, 7; of these last, 4 were males and 3 females; one, a male, had been bedridden for 1 year, and one, a female, for 7 years.

OUT-OF-DOOR EXERCISE.—Forty-five returns; bedridden, 7;

none, 16; of these, one 'can walk very well,' another 'stays in bed in cold weather;' little, 9; one of these 'mended the thatch of her cottage at 96, and was always the first home from church, being a rapid walker;' moderate, 1, she 'goes to church twice on Sundays;' eight walk out; of these, one 'walked four miles yesterday;' another 'walks daily half a mile, can walk three miles;' another is 'fond of sawing firewood;' two still work, one of these 'attended Hexham market, two years ago;' one 'worked in field at 102;' one was 'much out.'

SMOKES.—Forty-five returns; much, 7, four of these were women; little, 2, one was a woman; moderate, 3, one was a woman; none, 32; chews tobacco 1.

SNUFF.—Forty returns; none, 37; much, 1, this a woman who also smoked a little; little, 2, one being a woman, who did not smoke, the other a man, who smoked a little.

SLEEP.—Forty-four returns; good, 32; bad, 5; moderate, 7. *Number of Hours.*—Twenty-nine returns; average, rather more than $8\frac{1}{2}$ hours; 3 sleep 12 hours; 8 sleep 10 hours; 1 sleeps 4 hours; and 2 sleep 6 hours.

HOUR OF GOING TO BED.—Thirty-five returns; average, about 9 o'clock, one retires at 12 o'clock, one at 11, and 5 at 7 o'clock; 7 are bedridden.

HOUR OF RISING.—Thirty-five returns; average, about 8 o'clock; six rise at 6 o'clock, one at 5 o'clock, nine at 10 o'clock, one at 11 o'clock, and one at 4 P.M.

CHEST-GIRTH IN INSPIRATION. *Male.*—Six returns: average, $36\frac{1}{4}$ inches. *Female.*—Nine returns; average, nearly 31 inches. Male and female together, average about 33 inches.

CHEST-GIRTH IN EXPIRATION. *Male.*—Five returns; average, about $36\frac{1}{8}$ inches. *Female.*—Seven returns; average, nearly 30 inches. Male and female together, average about $32\frac{1}{2}$ inches.

ELASTICITY OF RIB-CARTILAGES. *Male.*—Six returns; distinct, 1; indistinct, 5. *Female.*—Thirteen returns; distinct, 5; indistinct, 8.

PULSE.—Twenty-nine returns; average, 74—75 per minute. In some cases disease of the heart or lungs was returned, and in others the pulse-rate was unusually high and the condition of the heart and lungs was not detailed; excluding these cases, eleven in number, the average becomes 69—70 per minute. *Regular, Irregular, Intermittent.—* Twenty-eight returns; R. 24; Irr. 1; Int. 3. *Large, Small, Moderate.*—Twenty-seven returns; L. 9; S. 17; M. 1. *Compressible, Incompressible.*—Twenty-eight returns; C. 24; I. 4.

ARTERIES. *Male.*—Nine returns; even, 4; knotty, 2; tortuous and knotty, 1; tortuous, visible, and even, 2. *Female.*—Twenty returns; even, 8; tortuous, visible, and knotty, 3; visible and tortuous, 2; tortuous, visible, and even, 1; visible and even, 2; tortuous and knotty, 1; tortuous, 2; tortuous and even, 1.

ARCUS SENILIS. *Male.* Seven returns; much, 4; little, 1; absent, 2. *Female.*—Nineteen returns; much, 5; little, 8; absent, 6.

RESPIRATION. — Twenty-four returns; average, 24 per minute. Excluding those cases, eleven in number, in which heart or lung-disease was returned, or in which the rate of respiration was high, and the condition of the heart and lungs was not mentioned, the average becomes 21—22 per minute. *Regular and Irregular.*—Twenty-four returns; regular, 21; irregular, 3.

TEETH.—Forty-two returns; 24 had none. In 13 the teeth were specified; amongst these 13 cases, there were 144 teeth: upper jaw, 63—incisors, 19; canines, 8; molars, 36:

lower jaw, 81—incisors, 23; canines, 13; molars, 45.   In five cases the number was alone given.   Average (42 cases) 4—5 teeth.   In one case, they 'all came out whole.'   *Males.*—Fourteen returns; 6 had none; average 4 teeth.   *Females.*—Twenty-eight returns; 18 had none; average, nearly 5 teeth.   Three females had complete sets, and one had 17 teeth; one male had 24, and another 16 teeth.

ARTIFICIAL TEETH.—Thirty-eight returns; none, 34; yes, 4; 1 (female); many years, 2 (male and female); from 50—90, 1 (female).

EVIDENCES OF FAILURE.—Thirty-five returns; none, 18; failures in 17 cases.   *Heart*, 2.—In one, 'sounds distinct, no murmur, very irregular, at one minute beating 60—70, and at another double as fast;' in the other, 'circulation feeble, frequently sick and faint, as if she were going.'   *Heart and Lungs*, 3.—In one, 'heart and lung-sounds weak;' in another, 'pulse intermits 6 times in minute, impulse weak, slight bronchitis;' in another, 'aortic regurgitation, slight bronchitis.'   *Heart and urinary organs*, 3.—In one, 'loud systolic *bruit* at base, no appreciable interference with circulation, micturition frequent;' in another, 'heart-sounds tumultuous and irregular, micturition frequent;' in another, 'heart's action slightly irregular, this not discernible in the pulse, frequent micturition.'   *Lungs*, 2.—In one, 'chronic bronchitis;' in the other, 'cough for four months.'   *Brain*, 3.—Senile dementia in two cases, one of these 'childish for 6 years;' in the third case, apoplexy, right hemiplegia, aphasia, and death shortly after.   *Brain and Urinary*, one 'Aphasia for 14 days, incontinence of urine.'—One had 'some incontinence for 10 years;' in two others, micturition was slow; and in another, 'incontinence.'

MICTURITION. *Male.*—Ten returns; natural, 7 ; slow, 2 ; frequent, 1. *Female.*—Twenty-three returns; natural, 18; frequent, 2; incontinence, 3—in one case for 10 years.

PAST HISTORY.

AGE WHEN MARRIED. *Male.*—Twelve returns; average, nearly 23 years. *Female.*—Nineteen returns; average, nearly 25 years.

DURATION OF MARRIED LIFE. *Male.*—Twelve returns; average, 54–55 years. *Female.*—Eighteen returns; average, 53–54 years.

NUMBER OF CHILDREN. *Male.*—Sixteen returns; average, 6–7 children. *Female.*—Twenty-one returns; average 6 children. One male and one female had no children.

FIRST, OR—CHILD OF PARENTS.—Thirty-eight returns; average, about third child. Twelve were 'first children,' and of these 2 were also the 'only children.' In 14 cases the number of the family was also returned, averaging seven.

AFFLUENT, COMFORTABLE, POOR.—Forty-nine returns; A, 3 ; C. 28; P. 18.

STOUT, SPARE, AVERAGE.—Forty-seven returns; St. 3 ; Sp. 28; A. 16.

DELICATE, ROBUST, AVERAGE.—Forty-three returns; D. 2; R. 28; A. 13.

HEALTH.—Forty-five returns ; good, 45.

AILING.—Twenty-one returns; rarely, 19; often (male) 1 ; never, 1.

DIGESTION.—Forty-five returns; good, 44 ; indifferent, 1.

BOWELS.—Forty-two returns; good (daily), 34; costive, 6 ; alternate days, 1 ; relaxed, 1.

BALDNESS.—Eighteen returns; late, 14; early, 3; none, 1.

GREYNESS.—Forty-two returns; late, 29; early, 12; none, 1.

DISPOSITION.—Forty-three returns; placid, 14; irritable, 4; energetic, 10; irritable and energetic, 8; placid and energetic, 7.

INTELLECT.—Forty-six returns; average, 32; high, 10; low, 4.

HABITS.—Forty-eight returns; active, 46; moderate, 2.

OUT-OF-DOOR EXERCISE.—Forty-one returns; much, 27; little, 6; moderate, 8.

HOURS IN BED.—Twenty-nine returns; average, 7 hours; one also returned as 'few hours.'

HOUR OF RISING.—Thirty-three returns; average, about 6 o'clock; one also returned as 'late.'

SLEEPER.—Forty-three returns; good, 38; average, 5.

APPETITE.—Forty-three returns; good, 42; indifferent, 1.

EATER.—Forty-one returns; average, 27; small, 7; large, 7.

ALCOHOL.—Forty-one returns; none, 12; moderate, 8; little, 20; and one who 'always drank as much as I could, and always will do,' *vide* also remarks on Nos. 8, 14, 35 (p. 53).

ANIMAL FOOD.—Thirty-five returns; moderate, 7; little, 28.

SMOKE. *Male.*—Fifteen returns; much, 7; little, 1; none, 7. *Female.*—Twenty-eight returns; much, 4; little, 1; moderate, 1; none, 22.

SNUFF. *Male.*—Fifteen returns; none, 13; 'yes,' 2. *Female.*—Twenty-three returns; none, 21; 'yes,' 1; much, 1.

CHAPTER IV.

REPORTS OF ADDITIONAL CENTENARIANS.

ACCOUNT OF NINETEEN ADDITIONAL CENTE-
NARIANS, MAKING THE ENTIRE NUMBER
SEVENTY-ONE.

THE following reports of nineteen centenarians were
received subsequently to the publication of the analyses
and resumé of the fifty-two given in the preceding chapter.
I have thought it best to keep them separate that it may
be seen how far they are confirmatory of the results given
in that chapter.

The women—ten to nine—are still in excess of the
men, though the proportion is not quite so great as we
found before.

The good health and vigour, bodily and mental, and
the happiness attaching to the centenarian period are no
less remarkable than we before noticed. In one only are

the digestion and appetite said to be indifferent; and in one only was there any evidence of gouty or rheumatic affection of the finger-joints. Fourteen enjoyed good sight, though some used glasses, and one had done so for more than forty years. In ten hearing was good. In three the sight is reported as indifferent; and this is said of the hearing in five. The mental faculties and the memory are generally well preserved. In three the intelligence is said to be 'high,' in five to be 'good,' and in six to be 'average'; and nothing is more interesting and satisfactory than to observe how often the words 'cheerful,' 'cheery,' 'chatty,' 'amiable,' 'good tempered,' 'placid,' and 'energetic' are applied to them. No. 68 "makes no trouble of nothing;" No. 53 retained her faculties till within a few days of her death, which was caused by no special disease but was from sheer old age; No. 54 danced on her 101st birthday; No. 59 supports himself by cleaning a chapel, and walks a mile each way every morning to fetch milk for the minister; No. 63 gives no evidence of failure; No. 65 is "wonderfully bright and cheerful, and had not long come in from chopping wood in the woodhouse;" No. 69 "transacts his own business and looks after his houses and other property and visited his native village last summer, and means to live another twenty years if he can;" No. 70 could thread a needle and had keen memory and good intellect to the last. Excellent specimens are these of the conservation of energy in the centenarian frame. The good state of the arteries and the elasticity of the chest-walls are mentioned in some. In the one woman and the seven men, in the cases of whom it is mentioned, micturition is said to be natural; and it would probably have been mentioned if it had not been so in the others.

The average height of the four women of whom it is given is 5 ft. 3 in., and of the six men, omitting No. 59, is 5 ft. 5 in., this being scarcely equal to that of those on our list and therefore not quite so confirmatory of Mr Roberts's observations (p. 112).

The remarks at p. 41 respecting the longevity of 'first children' are fully confirmed by the fact that five of this number were first children. Moreover we have another instance (No. 55) in which one of the parents was a 'twin.' The productive capacity is again well evinced by the fact that of the seven women who were married six had respectively eight, five, two, twelve, nine and eleven children. In the seventh the number of the children is not given; but it is stated that three of her children are still alive. One of the men had ten children, another twelve, and a third twenty-nine. There is therefore fair prospect of the maintenance, rather the increase, of the centenarian quality by inheritance.

Confirmatory evidence of what has been said respect-

H. C.   5

ing the teeth is afforded by their complete absence in
seven of the women and in two of the men. Six had
respectively 4, 4, 10, 'a few,' 8 and 6; and these were
chiefly in the lower jaw.

The average rate of the pulse in the nine persons
in whom it is given amounts only to 63, whereas that
deduced from the former list is 74; in No. 71 who was in ʿ
a very feeble state it was 92. The average in the cases
here given is probably brought below the normal by No. 57,
in whom the pulse was only 54, and still more by No. 68, in
whom it was only 42, although this was apparently no indication of failure in the latter, for he was able to walk up
moderately high hills, better even, it is said, than he could
walk down them, the latter performance being interfered
with by the presence of corns. In four the pulse is said to
intermit and in five to be regular. In these persons again
very little evidence is given of degenerative changes in the
arterial walls. In one only are they said to be granular.
The chest expansion during inspiration in the six in whom
it is given amounts to nearly an inch, which is rather
greater than that stated in the analysis of the former list.

We read in these centenarians only of 'good,' 'excellent' or 'vigorous' health throughout life, with good
appetite and digestion, a great immunity from illness and
maladies, a placid cheerful energetic disposition, good
mental power and active life. Indeed those of whom

the account is here given seem on the whole to have enjoyed even a higher level of health and strength throughout life than those from whom the report in the former chapter was made; and they were also even more remarkable for their temperance in eating and drinking.

Several are members of long-lived families; but the father of No. 57 is said to have died at 44 of consumption.

The recovering power from illness in the aged is evinced in Nos. 54, 62 and 70; and No. 57 is said to have been confined to bed by debility for two years between sixty and seventy. No. 60 rallied in a wonderful way from attacks of bronchitis, to one of which she ultimately succumbed; and No. 62 in like manner rallied from pneumonia four months before death. Nos. 67 and 68 had severe fever (typhoid) between fifty and sixty.

The following are the cases referred to.

53. Dr Selby, of Portwilliam, writes: " Died at Portwilliam, Wigtonshire, on December 29th, 1886, Betsy Boath—married name Stirling; born May 18th, 1784; married and had eight children, who predeceased her; first child born in 1810, when she was 26 years of age. A brother of hers died in April, 1885, and there were between her and him a sister who died two years since, aged 89 years, and another three years since, aged 91 years. She was born in Kennettles, Forfarshire, and

5—2

lived in that part of the country till May, 1860, when she removed to this place. She was always a very healthy woman, quiet and industrious, and very temperate in her habits. She retained her faculties to within a few days of her death, and could read with the aid of spectacles. She was confined to bed for a fortnight at the last, and died of no special disease, but of sheer old age."

54. Dr Smith, of Pershore, sends the following account of Sarah White, a widow, who died at Pershore eight years ago, aged 101; was strong and stout, about 5 feet, and erect; was in a comatose state at 99 for some weeks after a chill from sitting in a draught, but recovered, and danced and sang on her 101st birthday; joints natural; digestion and appetite good; toothless; hearing and sight indifferent; was intelligent, with good memory, and good-tempered; in moderate circumstances; had five children; had been an early riser, and drank some beer; did not smoke or take snuff.

55. Dr Smith also reports of Sarah Mumford, a widow, who had had ten children, that she died, aged 103, of diarrhœa, at Pershore; was about 5 feet; a brisk, energetic, sociable, intelligent person, but childish at last; good hearing, sight, digestion, and appetite; toothless; took little alcohol; was able to walk about; always a very abstemious person, taking very little meat, not smoking or chewing tobacco; had no illnesses, ailments, or accidents,

indeed always good health; was the first child of her parents, one of whom was a twin. Three of her children are alive, aged 67, 70, and 75.

Dr Smith attended both the above.

56. Dr Cameron, of Bawtry, sends me the following account of Jane Neale, a widow, born May 17th, 1785, who died September 8th, 1885. She was in church, and received the Communion on her 100th birthday, which happened on a Sunday; was confined to bed for two months, and sank very gradually. She resided at Bawtry in comfortable circumstances; of average general condition; used glasses, but had good sight, hearing, digestion, and appetite, and regular action of bowels, rarely taking medicine; of energetic character, high intellect, and with good memory; active; a good sleeper, going to bed about 10, and rising between 7 and 8; no teeth, natural or artificial; slight deformity of finger-joints; pulse 72, regular, large, compressible; little arcus senilis; micturition natural; had two children; two sisters died at the age of 86.

57. Dr Sinclair, of Kirkwall, sends me the following note, of Robert Yorston.—Born December 10th, 1786 (register in family Bible); poor, spare and feeble, lately confined to bed by weakness, but contented, pleased to see friends and still able to shave himself; voice full; hearing and sight indifferent, used glasses many years; finger-joints

natural; digestion and appetite good; small eater, four
meals, ½ ounce whisky at night, very little meat; bowels act
irregularly, and he often takes an aperient; is of placid
disposition, has full possession of his mental faculties, and
has fair memory; no maladies; micturition natural; four
lower incisors remain; rather under middle height; youth-
ful look; chest-girth, 37 inches in inspiration, 36 in expiration; elasticity of rib-cartilages distinct; pulse 54,
regular, large, incompressible; arteries even; respiration
24, regular; arcus senilis much; no evidence of failure
in great organs. He worked as a shoemaker till 90, at
Kirkwall; was married at 28, and had 12 children; was
the first child of two; was a spare man, always had good
health, digestion, and regular action of bowels, of cheerful,
placid disposition, average intellect, active, but took little
out-door exercise; rose at 7, good sleeper, good appetite
but small eater, no alcohol and very little meat; no
tobacco; when between 60 and 70 was in bed two years
from debility, gradually recovered. His father was 33
when Yorston was born, and died at 44, of phthisis. His
mother died at 89, and his sister at 65, of cancer of intestines. Six of his twelve children are alive, ages from
48 to 71; one died of locomotor ataxy aged 68, another
of dropsy aged 48, and others when young. No blood-
relationship between his parents.—He died July 8, 1888,
quietly and painlessly after a period of weakness but

without illness. Had been confined to bed between two and three years.

58. C. Ogden, M.R.C.S., of Rochdale, writes of Robert Brearley, who was born May 20th, 1787, whose baptismal certificate is dated June 10th, 1787, and who is in comfortable circumstances, that he is of average condition, erect, 5 feet 6 inches, active and walks about; has seen him walking out this winter, one cold, foggy, very trying morning; has clear full voice, good hearing, used glasses for thirty years, but cannot read now; finger-joints natural, teeth all gone; good digestion, appetite, and action of bowels; is a moderate eater, takes no alcohol, but a moderate amount of meat; energetic and placid; average intellect, good memory; goes to bed at 9, gets up at 11; has no maladies; micturition natural; chest-girth 37 inches in inspiration, 36 in expiration; elasticity of rib-cartilages distinct; pulse 70, regular, small, incompressible; arteries visible and even; respirations 20, regular; arcus senilis little; no evidence of failure in great organs.—He was a flannel-weaver; was a first child; married at 22, wife lived 49 years after, and had three children; was always in comfortable circumstances; was stout; good health, appetite and digestion, action of bowels, and sleep; was active, walked many miles and used to hunt on foot; got up at 4 or 5; an average eater, moderate animal food, very little alcohol, no tobacco; of

average intellect; had few ailments; his father's father
died aged 65, mother aged 35; mother's mother at 74;
father 54, mother 85; brother 79, sisters 86 and 80; one
child is alive, aged 75, one died at 65 of dropsy and
another, aged 25, of rupture of blood-vessel.

59. A. W. Steer, M.R.C.S.E., of Stewart Town, Jamaica, sends me the following account of a native man,
named Tawny, supposed to be 115, who was given as a
wedding present to Mr Steer's great-grandparents at their
wedding in 1783; and it is not the custom to make a
present of a slave till he is developed into useful property,
varying from 12 to 16. Quite' black; grey, woolly hair;
supports himself by cleaning a chapel, and walks a .mile
each way every morning, to fetch milk for the minister.
Came to Mr Steer's wedding a few months ago to give
good wishes, as he has been to all the weddings in the
family for four generations; is 5 feet high, weight about
90 pounds; spare, erect, of average strength; active and
energetic; muscles well developed; clear voice; good sight,
hearing, appetite, digestion, and sleep; moderate eater,
two meals, little animal food; never tasted alcohol; joints
natural; average intellect and good memory; 50 years of
married life, two children, and one of these is quite an old
man; was a first child, always had good health; employed
in slave work, and got up at daylight; no illness, ailments,
or accidents since boyhood. Two of his sisters are alive,

one aged 80, the other a little younger than himself. His father was a native of Jamaica, his mother an African; chest-girth in inspiration 31½ inches, expiration 31, elasticity indistinct; pulse 62, regular and small; arteries tortuous; respirations 15, regular; much arcus senilis; 10 teeth: 2 incisors, 1 canine, 4 molars in upper jaw, 1 incisor and 2 molars in lower; heart sounds clear and distinct; micturition natural; temperature in rectum 98·4°.

60. H. C. Smith, M.R.C.S., of Notting Hill, enclosed baptismal certificate of his aunt, Miss Annie Spurr, of whom he saw much in the latter part of her life. She died aged 104 (born March, 1777, died in 1881), was the first child of her parents, was about 5 feet 5 inches, no gouty affection of hands, a self-sacrificing, truly religious person, had good health, used spectacles late in life only for reading, deaf.—Kept ladies' school for sixty years; retained her faculties till death; broke the neck of the thigh bone three years before death, and unable to walk afterwards. Latterly had slight attacks of bronchitis, but always rallied in a wonderful way; sank at last after a slight attack, with gradually increasing insensibility. Her father, a German, died at 75, her mother, English, at 68. Was cheerful, amiable, interested in what was going on in the world, and retained her faculties with little change till about a year before death.

61. A relative sends, through Sir Dyce Duckworth,

the account of Miss Catherine Heathorne, who lived, at Maidstone, to 103; 5 feet 2 inches, bent, glasses twenty years, joints natural, no teeth, natural or artificial, high intellectual powers, plenty of out-door exercise, an early riser, average sleeper, able to reinvigorate herself by a short nap, good appetite, average eater, little alcohol, no illnesses; the fourth child of fifteen ; long-lived family.

62. Dr Kenny, of Dublin, sends report of William Holland, aged 104, in the Union Hospital. Widower, formerly sailor and day labourer; 5 feet 1 inch; average strength; uses glasses; good hearing; finger-joints natural; good appetite and digestion, moderate eater, two meals, a little whisky, regular bowels, placid disposition, average intellect; active, walks about; cheerful and chatty, some rheumatic pains.—Was a sailor and a servant, poor, always spare and healthy, bald and grey late, an early riser, good sleeper, good appetite, average eater, and moderate drinker; had attack of pneumonia four months before death, from which he had recovered when an attack of diarrhœa carried him off in two days. Pulse about 64, regular, rather large and compressible; a few teeth remained; micturition slow but natural; some evidence of aortic disease in the last few years. Dr Kenny remarks that the recovery from pneumonia showed the soundness of his organs, and that the attack was a good example of the insidious manner in which that disease comes on in old age.

63. Mr Nicoll, a medical student of Peterhouse, reports of John Ronan, living in Dunowth, co. Cork, that he is reported to be 104, was married at 40; his wife lived 52 years with him, and bore ten children; that he is strong, and walks about; 5 feet 8 inches, 11 stone, erect, of average strength, tough as an oak, good sight and hearing, finger-joints natural, eight teeth remaining (one upper canine, four lower incisors, two canine, one molar), good appetite and digestion, three meals, seldom alcohol, placid disposition, very shrewd, fair memory, good sleep, goes to bed about 8, gets up about 12; was a ·farm labourer, had good health, got up at 5; average eater, took alcohol when he could get it, which was seldom; lived much on fish, smoked much; had fever about 40; pulse 72, intermitting, large, incompressible; arteries even; respiration 24; arcus senilis little; no evidence of failure, micturition quite natural.

64. Professor Chiene, of Edinburgh, sends the account given by Mr Bowman of Crail, of Mrs Murray, whom he, at the age of 18, was taken to see when she was 100, as she wished to see the seventh John Chiene in lineal succession. She was born at Kilduncan in 1761, and died August 1st, 1862, having broken her thigh-bone by a fall in walking across her room several weeks previously; had nine children, all of whom, with one exception, reached maturity. She lived alone, under the care of an old and

faithful servant; took a daily short walk out-of-doors till her accident; had good sight with spectacles, fair hearing; was quite clear-headed, always cheery. It was easy to maintain conversation with her, and she would respond with a hearty laugh to anything humorous; very tidy and particular in her dress; employed herself busily in knitting, and did it excellently, although disadvantaged by the contraction of the third and fourth fingers of each hand, which were doubled into the palm. Teeth had long been gone, but her splendid health was not affected thereby; and to the last distinct traces remained of the beauty for which, in her youth, she had been distinguished.

65.   A. D. Rolleston, of St Bartholomew's Hospital, sends note of Thomas Thatcher, 7, Crown Court, Warwick Lane, E.C., aged 100, poor, bent, loud clear voice, good sight and hearing, joints natural: one upper molar tooth and below two incisors, two canine, and one molar; little arcus senilis; appetite bad, takes a little rum; average intellect; moderate memory; good sleep; had no illnesses.

66.   The Rev. F. Howlett, and W. Curtis, M.R.C.S., send accounts from which the following is taken of William Bone, in his 100th year, who still acts, and has done so for sixty years, as parish clerk; though very deaf for twelve years, has good sight (using glasses for about ten years), loud clear voice and good health, with moderate digestion and appetite, a moderate eater, taking little

meat and alcohol; daily action of bowels; no teeth; chest-
girth 33½ in inspiration, 32¾ in expiration; elasticity of
rib-cartilages distinct; pulse 80, occasionally intermitting,
large and compressible; arteries visible, but without knottiness; respirations 22, and regular; much arcus senilis;
heart, lungs, brain, urinary, and other organs healthy;
micturition natural; a large inguinal rupture being his
chief trouble. He is 5 feet 7 inches, weighs 10 stone,
somewhat bent, active, with good intellect and memory;
a moderate sleeper, goes to bed at 9, and rises at 7.30. A
tailor and gardener, in comfortable circumstances, and
kept a public-house from 1812 to 1819, but was always
very temperate in eating and drinking; good appetite
and digestion, and average eater; rose before 5; was a
first child; lived at East Tisted; married at 24, for thirty-
three years, and had six children; described as of high
intellect, active, and energetic, though placid; had always
good health; no illnesses, accidents, or ailments, except
occasional slight erysipelas in the face and legs. His
mother lived to 100, and her parents to a great age. His
father died at 60, and his parents were not long-lived.
Mr Curtis describes him as "wonderfully bright and
cheerful, and had not long come in from chopping wood
in the wood-house." According to a certificate in the
Parish Register he entered his 101st year on Oct. 3, 1887;
and on that day was present at a congratulatory meeting

of the parishioners, walked up a steep lane, and chimed
three church bells all at once without assistance, in
honour of the Queen's Jubilee and his birthday.

67.   Dr O'Connor, of Chatteris, writes of Mary Pidley,
æt. 100; date of birth, in family Bible, Feb. 14, 1787, of
marriage, 1808. She is poor, rather full blooded, of average
stoutness and strength; 5 ft. 1 in.; 8 stone; erect; with clear
full voice; short sight, needing glasses; indifferent hearing;
hands natural; no teeth; digestion good; appetite moderate; 4 meals daily; no alcohol; little meat; bowels
irregular; often takes aperients; placid disposition; average
intellect; memory good for past events; confined to bed
but no malady; chest-girth 28 in inspiration and 27 in
expiration; elasticity of chest-wall indistinct; pulse 60,
regular, moderate, compressible; arteries even; inspiration
15, regular; no arcus senilis; micturition slow; heart's
sounds natural.—She was formerly a washerwoman; stout;
had always good health, though constipated; was grey
early; a placid person, of average intellect, active, much
out-of-doors, about 6 hours in bed; up at 5, often earlier;
had good appetite; an average eater, taking meat once
a day and a little beer, neither smoked nor took snuff;
was the ninth child of her parents; had severe typhus at
60, but no other illness; was married at from 20 to 80,
and had 12 children, of whom 5, from 60 to 73, are alive;
one died of phthisis; could give no further information

about her family except that there had been no blood-relationship.

68.　From E. Brickwell, M.R.C.S., of Sawbridgeworth, I have the following account of Susanna Whybrow, æt. 100 and 8 months. She is in comfortable circumstances; pale, rather fat, and of average strength; 5 ft. 4 in.; bent; loud clear voice; good sight, used glasses 20 years; good hearing; no teeth; good appetite and digestion; a moderate eater; takes a little beer and spirit and a little meat; bowels act daily, rarely takes aperient; of placid disposition and average intellect, with good memory for recent as well as past events; confined to bed two months but has no malady, though her state is weaker; takes snuff but does not smoke; sleeps well; chest-girth $30\frac{1}{2}$ in inspiration and $29\frac{1}{2}$ in expiration; elasticity of chest-wall distinct; pulse 64, intermitting, small, compressible; arteries granular; respiration 17, regular; much arcus senilis; heart's sound natural; micturition natural.—She was the sixth child; married to agricultural labourer at 19 for 69 years, and had 11 children; always had excellent health; was robust and of average stoutness; had good digestion and regular action of bowels; became grey late; was of placid dis-position, making "no trouble o'nothing, Sir"; was active; in bed 7 hours, up at 4 or 5; a good sleeper, with good appetite, an average eater, very little beer and little animal food; a snuff-taker, but not a smoker; had severe typhoid at 50, but no other ailment. Her mother's mother was 80, her father 80 and her mother 87, a brother 80; children 62, 73 and 75, uncertain about others; no blood-relationship between her parents.

69. I am indebted to H. Dew, M.R.C.S., of Bristol, for the following. Edward Grubb, aged 105 and 6 months, living in Bristol; strong, of average stoutness, neither full blooded nor pale; 5 ft. 5; 11 stone; erect, with loud clear voice; good sight, used glasses forty years; good hearing; no artificial teeth; finger-joints natural; has 4 teeth (one upper molar, below two incisors one canine and one molar); moderate digestion and appetite and moderate eater; four meals daily with half-pint of beer and 1½ oz. of whisky and ¼ lb. of meat; bowels irregular, but he does not take aperients; is energetic, of average intellect and good memory for past and recent events; active, walking 2 to 4 miles daily; takes snuff but does not smoke; sleeps well, 10 hours, and is 12 hours in bed; has no maladies; chest-girth 36½ inches in inspiration and 35 in expiration; elasticity of rib-cartilages distinct; pulse 48, regular and compressible; arteries even; respiration 20, regular; little arcus senilis; heart's sounds natural; no evidence of failure in any organ, and micturition natural.—Was a farm labourer in Hereford-shire; married from 30 to 85 years, but had no children; was the third child of his parents; a spare person, mode-

rately robust, always had good health, except that his digestion was indifferent and bowels irregular; became grey late; of energetic disposition and average intellect; much out; in bed about 6 hours; up at 5, a good sleeper; had good appetite, taking daily about ½ lb. of meat, two pints of beer and a glass of whisky; took snuff but did not smoke; no illness; nearly killed by a bull. Of his family he knows only that a sister is alive aged 97; no blood-relationship between his parents.

Dr Beddoe, of Bristol, has also been good enough to send me the particulars of Mr Grubb, which state that he is 105, and which, in most respects, correspond with those given by Mr Dew. He adds that he always shaves himself, and used to clean his windows inside and out and do his own cooking till five years ago when a niece came to live with him, and that he still transacts his own business and looks after his houses and other property. He describes his intellectual powers as 'high'; that he was 80 years old when gored by the bull; was ill for a month or two and was bled; that his father died at 35 after a short illness, and his mother at 102, also that another sister died at 80. He found elasticity of rib-cartilages distinct; the pulse 42, small and compressible, and remarks that though the pulse is so slow (he found it also irregular) the old man walks up moderate hills better than down, his corns interfering with the latter performance; very cheerful and lively, and says he means to live another 20 years if he can. Last summer visited his native village, but could not make out clearly when he was baptised. He retired from business 48 years ago, and "I have little doubt," Dr Beddoe adds, "that he is as old as he thinks or thereabouts."

70. The following interesting account of Peggy Walsh, reputed to have been 124 at the time of her death, is kindly sent by Miss Miller, of Milford, Hally Mount, co. Mayo, who says that "although there is no register of our dear old nurse's birth we fully believe her to have been 124 years old when she died in January 7, 1867. Comparing her age with that of our ancestors whom she nursed it could not be less." "For the last 40 years of Peggy's life she had lived with my mother, and to the very last her sight and hearing were perfect. She *never* used glasses and could thread a fine needle. Her memory of both past and recent events was very keen, and she retained her intellect to the last moment. She died after a few days' illness of a bronchial attack. She was one of the most amiable and sympathising women I ever met and very cheerful. We looked on her quite as a friend and missed her very much. Although she had no teeth for the 40 years she was with my mother, the want did not inconvenience her as she ate like everybody else." She was about 5 ft. 5, very light slight figure

and erect, with clear voice, good appetite and digestion, a moderate eater, taking 4 meals, meat at dinner, and about an ounce of whisky in water, never took aperients, bowels acting regularly. She was of placid disposition, energetic and high intellect, active, took a little snuff, a moderate sleeper; had a few attacks of bronchitis when above 100, not known to have previously suffered any maladies. Family history not known.

71. The following account has been kindly sent me by Dr Davidson, of Liverpool. See also *Brit. Med. Journal,* Feb. 23, 1889, p. 439.

Terence McArdle, 7 Court, Shaw Street, Liverpool, stated to be æt. 106, on 15th of last March, dock labourer, and latterly a salt-weigher. Born near Armagh. He says he was married at the age of 17, very soon after the Irish Rebellion (1798), which he remembers perfectly.

He had 15 children by his first wife, and 14 by his second wife, the youngest of whom is the only survivor, a woman aged 45, who now lives with him. (She is his 29th child, and her baptismal register is June, 1844—this has been verified.)

He came to Liverpool 81 years ago and worked till 2 years ago. For the last 10 or 11 months has been bedridden.

He says his paternal grandfather lived to the age of 110.

Mr Longbottom, manager of Messrs Holmes and Sons, salt merchants, for whom McArdle latterly worked,

"Has known McArdle fully 40 years. When he first knew him he would be apparently about 50 or 60. He was very robust and continued so, carrying sacks of corn, very heavy work. Latterly he worked as a salt weigher up till about 18 months ago. He was a very good-tempered man, of average intelligence." In proof of McArdle's age, Mr L. states he remembers one of McArdle's children (not the eldest) died 15 years ago, aged between 50 and 60; Mr L.'s mother-in-law was born near Armagh. She died 7 years ago æt. 80. She remembered McArdle, when she was a girl, as a married man with children. James Egan from Armagh died 7 years ago æt. 80. He too, according to Mr L., remembered McArdle as married and with children when he was a boy.

McArdle says he enjoyed good health generally, but had fever twice, once in Ireland and once in Liverpool; was always active, cheerful; smoked a good deal; not a teetotaller, drank whisky, but not regularly; took very little meat, living principally on potatoes, bread, bacon and such like.

Present Condition. Lies in bed very helpless. Skin dry. Joints not deformed. Extremely emaciated. Only speaks when spoken to. Conjunctivæ covered with sticky mucus; pupils contracted (he was taking a cough mixture containing paregoric). Sight good: he told the time by my watch held a foot off in a very poorly lighted room. Cannot lift legs, but has fair grasp with right hand.

Respiration uneven and rather noisy, with intervals of slower and quieter breathing (resembling slightly Cheyne-Stokes' respiration). Occasional short cough, but no expectoration. Resp. 30 per min. Auscultation showed sounds fairly good, but there were some coarse râles. Girth of chest at nipple 33 inches. Costal cartilages very rigid; still, respiratory movements chiefly thoracic.

Circulatory System. Pulse 92 (left radial much smaller than right), artery tortuous but not distinctly calcified. Heart beats strongly, low down, in 6th intercostal space, nearly an inch outside nipple line. Impulse strong and somewhat irregular, no murmur.

Digestive System. Teeth. Lower jaw, 2 central incisors much wasted, left canine wanting, left molars much decayed, right tricuspids and molars absent.

Upper jaw, all teeth absent except a few stumps and the right canine and molar.

Abdomen greatly retracted, so that aorta could be easily felt beating strongly. It appeared to take a great curve towards the right side.

The bowels act of themselves once in 3 to 7 days. *Urinary.* Passes water about twice in 24 hours. Gives notice to his attendants, and never wets the bed.

He is somewhat deaf. His speech is thick and difficult to understand (mainly owing to the state of his mouth). Memory pretty good[1].

The correspondent of the *Times*, January 1st, 1887, gives account of an interview, in Vienna, with Magdalene Tonza, who entered her 112th year on Christmas Eve, in full possession of her mental faculties; lost the last of her teeth 30 years ago, excellent appetite, eats meat minced, drinks a little beer, and hobbles about the room with the aid of a stick. Sixty years were spent in her native village, Wittengau, Bohemia (where she was born in 1775), 30 years in another village, and she was past 90 when she came to Vienna, 17 years ago. Her youngest surviving grandchild is 60.

Dr Coker, of Chicago, writes me word that he attended a lady, aged 106, who recently died in that city of cancer of the tongue. This is the only instance of death of a centenarian from malignant disease that I have heard of.

A friend writes that Mrs Covill, of Settrington (see page 42), died on December 20th, within two months of being 102, after a week's illness, of bronchitis; she

---

[1] Dr Davidson writes, Feb. 26, 1889, " McArdle died this day."

retained possession of her faculties to the very last; received the Holy Communion in the afternoon of the day on which she died, was quite collected, thanked the clergyman, and wished him good-bye. My friend saw her a month ago, when she was as well as usual in mind and body. Thus she was sound and cheerful to the last, had a short illness, and a quiet peaceful end, affording a typical example of the close of a centenarian life.

In some respects contrasting with this is the account sent me by Dr Boswell, of Saffron Walden, respecting Mr N. (No. 11 on my list), who, for five or six months, was visibly declining, became unable to walk upstairs, and for three or four months had sacral bedsore, though not confined to bed. His legs were swollen, and he had a sore similar to the bedsore on one heel. This healed under treatment and relief from pressure, though the discharge was very profuse. The sacral sore, however, got worse. On December 12th his housekeeper, hearing his bell ring, went to him and found him breathing heavily, and she could not rouse him. He remained insensible, with inability to swallow, contracted pupils, and general rigidity of muscles, till his death, December 15th. "Cerebral hæmorrhage was undoubtedly the cause of his death, though the bedsore would have proved fatal had he lived a little longer."

The following remarks are in a letter from R. G.

Daunt, M.D., Edin., of San Paulo, Brazil, who has interested himself much in the subject of longevity: "I have known not a few individuals who attained the age of 114 years, one that of 115, many that of 100, and now in this district of Campinos exists a still strong and active man, Joseph Joachim do Prado—of good family—who counts 107 years, and whose mother and maternal grandmother reached the years of 112 and 122, the mother dying from an accident. Macrobians (of all races) of 100 to 130 are not at all infrequent—well-authenticated cases. Even cases of deaths at 140 are known to have occurred, especially in the mountainous province of Minos Jeraes. I cited (in the *Medical Times*) the district of Santo Amaro, near the capital of this province, as remarkable for the longevity of its inhabitants. The climate of Santo Amaro is cold, and the horses and cattle—natives of the district—are small, like those of Scotland. From what my residence of forty-three years in the interior of this country has permitted me to observe, I think it perfectly unreasonable to doubt the possibility of the attainment of the age of 150 years. The facts of longevity are more frequent among individuals of a mixed race of whites and Indians, next among Africans, and lastly among whites. It is a curious fact that, of a number of immigrants from the Açores who came here about seventy years ago, very few died with less than 100 years, and others reached

105, 109, 114. The truth of such ages I could safely swear to[1]."

I may refer to "the physical condition of centenarians, as derived from personal observation in nine genuine examples," by Sir George Duncan Gibb, in the *Journal of the Anthropological Institute*, 1872. Of these, two were men, and seven were women. They appear to have had remarkably good health, and the enjoyment of mental and bodily faculties; and in eight there was "an entire absence of those changes which are usually observed in persons approaching the allotted period of threescore and ten." One had been imbecile from childhood, and an inmate of a workhouse for probably the greater part of her life.

The following are among many instances of centenarianism that have been sent me. Mr W. B. Morris, in his investigations in connection with the evidence of St Patrick having lived to 120, finds that Pére Albert de Montebello was born May 13th, 1689, entered the Company of Jesus 1706, and was present in the Church of Gésu August 7th, 1814, when the bull restoring the Company was read in the presence of Pope Pius VII.—Mrs Whitely, a reputed centenarian, who is said to have had twenty-four children, appeared before the guardians at Hull in

[1] Instances of extreme longevity among Negroes and American Indians are also given by Pritchard, Humboldt, and others.

good health, shewing considerable vigour and no impairment of intellect though her sight was dim; *Manchester Guardian,* March 3, 1887.—Mary Prince, in the Sheffield Workhouse, attained her 100th year on March 8, had eleven children, married a soldier, who died forty years ago, accompanied the regiment to the Peninsula, and was present at the battle of Waterloo, used no glasses or stick, has been an inveterate smoker at least half a century to her daughter's knowledge, earned her living by washing till she was 90; *Leeds Mercury,* March 12, 1887.—A paragraph in the *Scotsman,* March 14, 1887, says that Hugh Macleod, living near Ullapool, is 105, having been born in 1782, "is brisk, lively, and able apparently to weather a few more winters yet; and in the same parish are Mrs MacNihbe æt. 103 and Mrs Macdeny, born in 1795, therefore in her 92nd year, who had 13 children, and is quite active."—Professor G. Buchanan of Glasgow writes respecting Mrs Gibson, who died recently at the age of 102. Principal Caird calling on her when she was over a hundred, found her bright and chatty, and sat with her for more than an hour; when he took leave she said in her usual easy humour, "Indeed principal, you have been here long enough. If you stay any longer you will make your wife jealous of me." "Not bad for a centenarian," adds the Professor.—One of the most remarkable instances that I have read is that of Colonel G. Perkins, in the *Boston*

Sunday Herald, U. S. May 5, 1888, who was born in the same year as the Constitution, and attained the age of 100 that day, and was to have a reception in honour of it the following day. He is still in active business, treasurer of the Norwich and Worcester railway—of which he was one of the incorporators in 1836—draws his checks, and looks over the important business as keenly and as unerringly as ever, has firm step, alert movement, and "his general expression of interest and participation in this world's affairs all announce him young in heart if old in experience." "He is about six feet in height, as straight as a pine, and has never known anything about sickness by personal experience. He has been a worker all his days, and has taken good care of himself, paying attention to diet, exercise and rules of health." His wife is 90 years old; they have lived together 71 years, and have two children living. The following remarks deserve to be repeated as the supplement to the account of such a life. "'Is life worth living?' ask those to whom the world seems evil. Not every life, perhaps. That life which physical infirmity fills with pain, that which moral corruption makes joyless to itself and baneful to others, may well seem worthless or worse. Even that life prolonged far beyond the usual term, whose closing years are impotent and vacant, may seem far from enviable. But in the presence of our venerable friend the cynic and the pessimist stand abashed.

In his aspect are no visible tokens of decay. In his serene afternoon (for shades have not yet darkened to evening) of moderate exertion, bodily health and cheerful piety, he finds life pleasant still, and his usefulness continues and increases, as daily, with his advancing age, he becomes more conspicuous as an example of those virtues which adorn life and make it happy." In harmony with this view we find in Zechariah's prediction of the Holy City when it shall be "called a city of truth; and the mountain of the Lord of hosts the holy mountain" that not only shall the "streets of the city be full of boys and girls playing in the streets thereof," but also "there shall yet old men and old women dwell in the streets of Jerusalem, and every man with his staff in his hand for very age."

CHAPTER V.

POST-MORTEM EXAMINATIONS OF CENTENA-
RIANS: WITH REMARKS.

OF the *post-mortem* examinations of centenarians which have been recorded (they are unfortunately but few), the first and best known, so far as I am aware, is that[1] of Thomas Parr, aged 152 years and 9 months, made by Dr William Harvey, famous for his discoveries respecting the circulation of the blood, by command of the king (Charles I.). The body was muscular, the chest and forearms hairy, the hair being still black, but the legs without hair. Organs of generation healthy; penis not retracted or extenuated; testes sound and large, "so that it seemed not improbable that the common report was true, namely, that he did public penance, under a conviction for incontinence, after he had passed his 100th year; and his wife, whom he had married in his 120th year, did not deny that he had intercourse with her, after the manner of other hus-

---

[1] *Harvey's Works*, published by the Sydenham Society, p. 589. Harvey expresses no doubt about his age. In this more sceptical period we may fairly admit him to rank among the centenarians.

bands with their wives." The chest was broad and ample;
the lungs, nowise fungous, adhered, especially on the right
side, to the ribs; heart large, thick and fibrous, with considerable quantity of fat; cartilages of ribs soft and flexible; stomach and intestines and all the viscera sound;
kidneys healthy, with the exception of a few watery
cysts; no appearance of stone in them or in the bladder;
spleen very small, scarcely equalling one of the kidneys;
a good deal of fat about the mesentery, omentum and
kidneys; brain healthy, firm and hard to the touch.

He "had obsèrved no rules or regular time for eating,
was ready to discuss any kind of eatable that was at
hand; his ordinary diet consisting of sub-rancid cheese
and milk in every form, coarse and hard bread, and small
drink, generally sour whey. On this sorry fare, but living
in his home, free from care, did this poor man attain to
such length of days. ... He was accustomed to walk about,
slightly supported between two persons; had been blind
for twenty years, heard extremely well, understood all that
was said to him, answered immediately to questions, and
had perfect apprehension of any matter in hand; his
memory was, however, greatly impaired." "He was accustomed, even in his 130th year, to engage lustily in
every kind of agricultural labour, whereby he earned his
bread, and he had even then the strength required to
thrash the corn." His death was attributed to the change

from the pure air of Shropshire to that of London, and to the change of diet, incidental to a residence in the house of the Earl of Arundel, by whom he was brought to town and presented as a remarkable sight to his Majesty the king.

2. Dr James Keill gives, in *Phil. Trans.* XXV., 1706, an account of the death and dissection of John Bayles, of Northampton, reputed to have been 130. The oldest people remembered him to have been old when they were young. Of late decrepit and carried about. His diet was anything he could get; but he had not eaten meat for some years, and of late lived only on small beer, bread, butter and sugar. Pulse irregular and intermitting for some years before death; went to stool but once in ten or twelve days for some years before death. A little man; body emaciated; abdominal viscera pale; spleen small; kidneys and urinary passages sound; a few yellow grains of gravel in the right kidney; cartilages of sternum not harder than they usually are; ribs brittle. "Lungs attached even to the pleura." Heart large, thick and fat; diameter of aorta above two inches; the abdominal and iliac arteries for the greatest part cartilaginous. Bones of skull sound and good; a small ossification in dura mater, by the falx. Brain more solid and firm than usual; ventricles full of serum. Genitals, both testicles and penis, of large size. He had lost sight for some years,

but hearing was good till he died. "The greatest part of his blood was in his arteries, whereas generally in all dead bodies the veins are full." This is attributed to the loss of elasticity in the arteries; and to the same cause is attributed the dryness and the deficiency of the secretions in the old. The strong fibrous heart, the low stature, the largeness of the chest and goodness of the lungs are regarded as having had the greatest share in promoting the longevity.

3. In *Phil. Trans.*, XLIV., p. 528, 1747, is an account by Haller of the examination of a decrepit woman reputed to be 100. Tissues dry; costal cartilages not yet osseous. Aorta, together with large arteries, osseous and rough ; the aorta much dilated (5 inches 2 lines in circumference), with valves indurated and earthy. Twenty small stones in gall-bladder.

4. Dr J. Beddoe, of Clifton, informs me that he "assisted at the *post-mortem* of a woman, credibly reported to be aged 106, who died from a burn. Her costal cartilages were normal. There was no evidence of her having ever had a tooth, so entirely had the alveoli been absorbed. One of her kidneys was perfectly obsolete. She exhibited signs of extreme tight-lacing."

5. Sir G. Duncan Gibb (*Journal of Anthropological Institute*, July, 1875) gives the necropsy of Mrs Leatherlund, believed by him to have died at the age of 110.

She was 4 feet 9 or 10 inches, and body proportionately small. Skin yellowish brown; muscular development good; no decided emaciation; some fat over the chest and abdomen; cartilages of ribs cut through with the greatest ease; lungs healthy; heart a little large, rather soft and flabby, with slight covering of fat; its muscular structure, cavities and valves appeared healthy; arch of the aorta enlarged, measuring 4 inches in circumference at its commencement and $3\frac{1}{4}$ inches at its termination. An atheromatous patch the size of a silver threepence at the lower surface of the transverse portion, and a ridge of atheroma at the left part of the ascending portion; scarcely a trace of omentum; stomach and alimentary canal, liver and gall-bladder healthy; spleen small but healthy; kidneys soft and flabby, but, as well as the ureters and bladder, healthy; uterus, Fallopian tubes and ovaries small; thoracic and abdominal blood-vessels healthy. The larynx and the rings of the trachea were perfect and flexible.

The same author attached much importance to the good conformation of the larynx and the erect position of the epiglottis, facilitating the passage of air to and from the lungs.

6. The most complete account of the examination of a centenarian is given by Rolleston[1]. John Pratt, re-

---

[1] *Scientific Papers and Addresses*, I. 111. Mr Hussey of Oxford writes to me that there were some doubts about this man being so old as stated.

puted to be 107. Father died aged 75; mother, 104; grandmother, 110. Habits some way short of strictly temperate. Examination made thirty-two hours after death. One upper canine. Dura mater closely adherent to skull; well-nigh continuous tracings marked the position of the coronal and sagittal sutures. No exostoses on interior of skull. Canals for meningeal arteries deepened by bands of bone on either side; but there is no mention that the skull was thick, dense, or heavy. Indeed the relation of diploë, internal and external tables, were much as in an ordinary skull. Weight of brain, 43 ounces. [He mentions one from a woman aged 100, 45 ounces.] Convolutions rounded, and to some extent atrophied; the fissure of Rolando, and the fissure anterior to it, being especially wider and deeper than natural. Cavities of lateral ventricles somewhat enlarged; numerous amylaceous bodies on surface of corpus striatum. Body appeared emaciated, but there was a considerable layer of yellowish fat over the pectoral muscles. Muscles looked pale, but showed the usual characters of striated muscle with great clearness and distinctness. Costal cartilages cut with greatest ease, of brownish yellow colour, from oil in cartilage cells. Died of acute pleurisy. Much fluid in right pleura; apex of right lung the seat of chronic pneumonia. Had cough for some months before death. Heart much loaded with fat; atheroma of aorta opposite the edges of valves, and calcareous deposit; very little beyond this—only one patch. Liver, 43 ounces; much oil in its cells. No mesenteric glands visible; Peyer's glands merely black specks; but these, under microscope, showed the same turgescence and soundness as in younger persons. Haller notes the absence of mesenteric system in advanced years. Spleen small, weighing 2 ounces; capsule tuberculated. Concretions of uric acid abundant in pelvis and calices of right kidney, and in bladder. Right kidney, $2\frac{3}{4}$ ounces; left, $2\frac{1}{4}$; both lobulated, and with numerous cysts scattered over the surface. Ureters much dilated. Bladder hypertrophied with sacculi and fasciculated. Lateral lobes of prostate large, like Home's plate 2, in Vol. II. Pediculated growths, size of pea, projected from its third lobe into the urethra; orifices of its ducts large. Testes not to be detected, though epididymis easily recognised by examination through the scrotum. No spermatozoa in vesiculæ seminales or vasa deferentia.

7. A. Melis, aged 104, an ecclesiastic who lived in Sardinia, by Dr Luigi Berrutti, quoted by Rolleston. Good digestion, middle-size, strongly built; fond of pleasures of table and good wine; bled at various periods some hundred times; died of pneumonia in spite of three bleedings. Curly black hair, and teeth in perfect preservation. Body muscular and fat; costal cartilages quite ossified; diploë and sutures of skull disappeared; dura mater

7—2

beset with bony plates; basilar and vertebral arteries ossified, also incrustations on aortic valves, aorta, and many
of its branches.   Heart fat, its muscular tissue firm.
Splenisation of lungs and bronchitis.

8.   Dr Holyoke, aged 103 (quoted by Rolleston, from
his *Memoirs*, Boston, U.S., 1829), a physician who settled
in Boston, at the age of 21, in 1749, and scarcely left till
the time of his death, and who led a life of the greatest
temperance.   Costal cartilages ossified; lungs pigmented;
fat about heart; cysts in kidneys; widened cerebral fissures,
and hydrocephalus *in vacuo* which he had predicted from
the sense of fluctuation in his head.

Dr Carrol, of New Brighton, New York, kindly sends
me the following corrections and additions made by a
grandson of Dr Holyoke.   He died at the age of 100 and
7 months, lived at Salem, 14 miles from Boston.   Though
not immoderate he did not practise temperance, his custom
being to have a large glassful of 'rum toddy' mixed every
morning, which he sipped at odd times through the day.
In addition to which he took two or three glasses of wine
at dinner.   He was an habitual smoker, and seldom went
to bed before midnight.   Even in his latest years he
always ascended the stairs, which were not very steep,
two at a time.

9.   Some years ago, I made a hasty examination of a
woman, reported to be 103, who died in this town of

bronchitis. No certificate as to date of birth was obtainable, but there was incontrovertible evidence of her great age. My attention was directed chiefly to the skeleton. The cartilages of the ribs were soft and yellowish from impregnation with oil. The skull was thick and heavy, weighing 28½ ounces, although only one tooth—a lower incisor—remained and the alveolary processes of the maxillæ were in great measure absorbed. The other bones examined were remarkably light and porous. Thus the thigh-bone, though large for a woman, weighed only five ounces. The skull and thigh-bone are in the museum of the University; and the lightness of the latter is in remarkable contrast with the heaviness of the former. The brain was shrunken, the fissures between the convolutions being wide, and occupied by sub-arachnoid fluid— "hydrocephalus *in vacuo*." The DENSITY AND THICKNESS OF THE SKULL, which I have observed not infrequently in old persons (my *Treatise on the Human Skeleton*, p. 195), and which may be regarded as an ossification *in vacuo*, is probably, like the accumulation of fluid in the sub-arachnoid spaces of the brain, due to a diminished pressure on the tissues and the blood-vessels, consequent on the diminution of the size of the brain, which takes place in advancing years. In some instances, absorption from the exterior keeps pace, or more than keeps pace, with the addition to the interior. Then the skull becomes smaller, and, it may be, thinner as well as smaller. Hence, although in some aged people the skull retains its size, and becomes thicker and heavier, in others it becomes smaller, but of the ordinary thickness, and, in some, it becomes small and extremely thin and light. In some cases, the external absorption takes place unequally, causing especially thinness at certain parts of the calvarium. This is peculiarly the case in the parietal bones on either side of the sagittal sutures; oval symmetrical, or nearly symmetrical, depressions being here formed, as though the outer and middle tables had been planed or chiselled off. In one specimen in the Cambridge Museum, the absorption had extended quite through the parietal bone at one part. I directed attention to these depressions in the parietals in my *Treatise on the Skeleton,* p. 242, and in the *Journal of Anatomy,* VIII., p. 136, but never could explain why the absorption should especially affect this particular region. Possibly the pressure of the occipito-frontalis tendon may have some relation to it. I may observe that the neck of the thigh-bone[1] in this old woman shows none of that lowering of the head and neck which is generally stated to occur, as a rule, in aged people, but which my observations[2] show very often, indeed generally, does not occur.

In the skeleton of a man, reputed to have died at the

---

[1] See photograph at the end of the book.
[2] See *Journal of Anatomy and Physiology,* XXIII. 273.

age of 105, which was shown by Professor Cunningham, of Trinity College, Dublin, at the meeting of the Anatomical Society in London, Feb. 6, 1889, the bones were so greasy that satisfactory maceration had not been obtained. The roughnesses of the long bones indicated that some deposit or growth on the exterior had continued, probably to the end of life. There were evidences of rheumatic arthritis, with much bony deposit, in various parts of the vertebral column and in some other joints. The costal cartilages, with the exception of a few earthy incrustations, were soft. The femur measured 17 inches, so that he had not been a very tall man. The upper part of the thigh-bone was of good size and form, and the angle formed by the neck with the shaft was 130. The skull was of fair size and moderate thickness.

One of the most interesting features in advancing age is the lessening size and weight of the CELL-MULTIPLYING AND BLOOD-PRODUCING ORGANS—THE SPLEEN, THE LYMPHATIC GLANDS, AND PEYER'S GLANDS—coincidently with the lessening of nutritive activity and therefore of the demand upon the blood-factors. These organs are, as we should expect, at their maximum in early life, when the growing and reparative work of nutrition is at its height, when the body is most increasing in size, and is most active in function. The thymus gland fades soon ; its special contribution, whatever it be, to the blood-compound, ceasing, as we may infer, to be required a few years after birth. The lymphatic glands are large in childhood and youth, and are easily excited to inflame, to enlarge unduly, and to take on other morbid conditions. As age advances, they become functionally and pathologically less active, and they are at their minimum in the centenarian. The mucous membrane of the stomach and intestines is usually thin and pale in the aged.

It is not a little remarkable that, whereas the greatest appreciable wasting is in the spleen and other organs which have relation to blood-making, the greatest increase is in the HEART which has relation to blood-propelling and which is, indeed, the chief agent in that work. This increase in the heart is not a little due to the accumulation of fat which often takes place upon it in advancing years, as well as to some thickening and other changes which affect its valves and fibrous tissues. Moreover, although the volume of the blood may be lessened in old age (and it does not appear that it always is so, for twenty-four of our centenarians are reported as full-blooded), the thickened, less elastic condition of the arteries, with the less perfect smoothness and evenness of their interior, renders the circulation of the blood a more laborious task for the heart, and causes some hypertrophy of its muscular structure.

The slight increase in the weight of the LUNGS observed

by Boyd in males is probably due to some thickening of their mucous and other tissues, associated with the lowered respiratory capacity which is caused, in great measure, by the diminished elasticity of the thoracic walls and of the lungs, and a consequent limitation of the respiratory range. This is evinced by the measurements of the chest-girth of our centenarians, which, on the average, do not show more than half an inch difference between inspiration and expiration (p. 58).

The degenerative changes in the ARTERIES—a substitution of fibrous, atheromatous or calcareous matter, for the elastic and muscular tissue, attended with thickening, dilatation and roughening—are less than might be expected. Though marked in Holyoke and Miles, and spoken of as a cartilaginous condition in Keill's case, they were confined to the commencement of the aorta in Rolleston's, and are not mentioned by Harvey. Of 29 returns in our analysis (p. 59), the arteries are reported "knotty" in 6, "even" in 18, and appear to have been large, tortuous or visible in 15. The loud systolic *bruit* in No. 13 (Mrs Covill) of our list indicated a roughening of the aorta, which was unattended with any obvious ill-effect; and the arteries were even, though tortuous and visible, in this person. There was nothing of the kind in the other two persons (12 and 23) whom I examined, and it is not mentioned in any of the other cases reported in the table, which possibly may be because attention was not specially directed to this point.

The CARTILAGES OF THE RIBS were ossified in Miles and Holyoke, but were as soft as natural in the cases reported by Harvey, Keill, Rolleston[1] and myself.

The BRAIN was found shrunken, with widened cerebral fissures, " hydrocephalus *in vacuo*," in Holyoke, also in the woman aged 103 examined by me. It was firm and hard in Parr and in Keill's case; and the convolutions were rounded and, to some extent, atrophied in Rolleston's. This shrinking of the brain, common in old age, and observed also in persons wasted by long illnesses, in habitual drinkers, and some others, is to be associated with the inability to maintain active and strong bodily and mental exertion, which, as our tables show, is commonly first manifested by fatigue, by weakening of memory for recent events, and is further manifested by impairment of control over emotions and thoughts and impulses as well as over bodily movements, and may go on to complete imbecility, with or without tremor or loss of muscular power, this last being usually first observed with regard to the urinary bladder.

The KIDNEYS were cystic in Parr, Holyoke, and Pratt,

---

[1] With reference to this, Rolleston (p. 153) remarks: "Old age causes very opposite changes to take place in bone; possibly it may act upon cartilages in equally differing ways."

and contained grains of sand in the last and in Keill's case. In Pratt the bladder was fasciculated, the prostate large and its ducts large, and pediculated growths projected from its third lobe. It will be observed that, out of 33 returns in the analysis (p. 61), the micturition is reported to be natural in 25. It is also stated to have been so in most of the cases the reports of which were subsequently received; and it is not stated to have been difficult or painful in any. All this is confirmatory of the observation that the prostatic and vesical affections, which cause the larger proportion of urinary troubles of advancing years in men, commonly manifest themselves about or before 70 in those who are predisposed to them, and do not, for the most part, permit the sufferers to attain to great age.

The following are taken from Dr Boyd's tables of the weights of the human body and of the internal organs[1].

He states (p. 261) that the average height of the adult male varies from 67·8 to 65 in.; of the female, from 63·2 to 61·6 in. The average weight of the adult male varies from 112·12 to 91·5 lbs.; of the female, from 95·2 to 76·9 lbs.

These examinations were made in 2086 cases in the St Marylebone Infirmary, and in 528 cases in the Somerset Lunatic Asylum; and he says they show a preponderance

[1] *Philosophical Transactions*, 1861.

in the insane male of 6 lbs., and in the female of 8 lbs., as compared with the sane. [This is probably due to the quiet and the good feeding in asylums.] Mr Roberts, in his letter in the *British Medical Journal* of January 1st, 1887, states that "the average stature and weight of English men and women of all classes is 5 ft. 7½ in. and 155 lbs. for males, and 5 ft. 2½ in. and 123 lbs. for females." This falls rather short of the average height of our centenarians, which is 5 ft. 8½ in. in males, and 5 ft. 3 in. in females (p. 56).

From the subjoined table taken from Boyd's paper it appears that, in persons above 80, the height and weight of the body remaining nearly the same (though in women, from whom the greater number of measurements were taken at above 80, there is a diminution in height and weight), the cerebral and the abdominal organs, including the kidneys, have wasted, whereas the thoracic organs have gained in weight; and the contrast between the wasting of the spleen, which has relation to blood-making, and the increase in the heart or blood-propelling organ, to which I have already alluded, is very marked.

From Boyd's Tables of the Average Weights of the Human Body and the Internal Organs.

	Sex.	Weight.		Height.		Encephalon.	Lungs.		Heart.	Stomach.	Liver.	Spleen.	Kidneys.	Pancreas.
		Lbs.	oz.	Ft.	ins.	Oz.	Right. Oz.	Left. Oz.	Oz.	Oz.	Oz.	Oz.	Oz.	Oz.
From 30 to 40 years	M	98	5	5	6·5	48·2	28·47	24·29	11·36	5·72	58·11	7·12	11·35	3·47
	F	87	0	5	2	43·09	18·74	17·04	9·45	5·34	53·61	6·13	10·34	3·05

Number examined, 103 males, 85 females.

	Sex.	Weight.		Height.		Encephalon.	Lungs.		Heart.	Stomach.	Liver.	Spleen.	Kidneys.	Pancreas.
Upwards of 80 years	M	99	0	5	6·7	45·34	30·46	24·30	12·1	4·99	41·01	4·27	8·25	2·83
	F	79	8	5	0	39·77	18·22	15·23	10·27	4·49	34·64	3·46	6·86	2·37

Number examined, 24 males, 75 females.

CHAPTER VI.

REPORT ON THE PRESENT CONDITION, HABITS, CIRCUMSTANCES, ETC., OF PERSONS AGED BETWEEN EIGHTY AND A HUNDRED.

THE following report, which relates to the present condition of the aged (that is, their condition at the time when the several reports were made), is founded upon the analyses of 824 persons printed at a subsequent page. Of these 824, 340 men and 282 women were between 80 and 90, and 92 men and 110 women were between 90 and 100.

Of the total number, 89 per cent. were, or had been, married; 48 per cent. were poor, 42 per cent. were in comfortable circumstances, and 10 per cent. only were described as being in affluent circumstances. This must not be regarded as representing the relations of poverty and affluence to longevity, because, in the first place, the poor, at all ages and in all districts, bear a large proportion to the affluent; and, secondly, our returns are largely made from the lower and middle classes, and, in many instances, from the inmates of union-workhouses, where a good number of aged people are found, and where information respecting them is most easily obtained.

The important questions of the relative longevity in different classes and among those following different occupations scarcely comes within the range of our inquiry. Indeed, they need carefully collected statistics of varying kinds, and much labour for their solution[1].

It does not appear that the Shakespearian sequence of the "lean and slippered pantaloon" to that of the "fair round judge" is by any means the ordinary one, for the 'spare' condition and the 'average' condition between 'spare' and 'fat' greatly predominate in our old people at all ages between 80 and 100. The 'average' condition is noted in 47 per cent. of the whole number, the 'spare' in 41 per cent., and the 'fat' only in 11 per cent.[2]; and the accounts of their condition at earlier periods of life indicate the same, by the far larger proportion having throughout life come under the denomination of 'spare' or 'average.'

The average HEIGHT of the men (67 inches), and of the

[1] See Class-Mortality Statistics, by Dr Grimshaw, *British Medical Journal*, August 13th, 1887; and Influence of Easy Circumstances on Longevity, by Dr Drysdale, *Ibid.*, August 20th.

[2] The round numbers only in the percentages and not the decimals are given, in most instances, which will account for the slight discrepancies occasionally observable, such as above, where $47 + 41 + 11 =$ only 99, instead of 100.

women (62 inches), if we take into account the lowering
of stature attendant upon age, which may be estimated at
not less than 2 inches, gives a high standard, the average
height of Englishmen at 25 being 67½ inches, and of
Englishwomen 62 inches.   This, as in the case of the centenarians (p. 56), corroborates the observations of Mr
Roberts (*British Medical Journal*, January 1st, 1887), who
found, " on grouping the measurements of a large number
of individuals together, that the curve of stature continued
to increase up to the age of 70, which was the limit of
the statistics;" and he expresses the opinion that "this
increasing stature of the population throughout life was
due to the greater viability of persons whose stature was
up to or above the average; or, in other words, to' the
weeding out by disease of the smaller and worst developed
members of the community."

The lowering of stature attendant upon age is due
partly to the loss of elasticity of the invertebral substances
and other parts of the frame, but chiefly to the inability
to attain and maintain the fully erect attitude, which
requires a certain effort on the part of the extensor
muscles, especially those of the knees and hips, an effort
which is fatiguing at all periods of life, and which cannot
be successfully made in the case of many aged persons.
A lowering of the heads of the thigh-bones, owing to an
alteration in the angle of the neck with the shaft, is,

according to my observations, less and of less common occurrence than is generally supposed. Indeed it need not enter into computation as a cause affecting the stature of the aged or as inducing the liability to fracture of this part in old persons. The fair maintenance of elasticity and erectness, shown in our list to be one of the attributes of great age, may lead us to infer that the lowering of stature in our old people had taken place to a less extent than is usual; and I have accordingly estimated it at not more than two inches.

The importance of this relation between physical development and longevity acquires increasing force in proportion to the value of the evidence which is being adduced as to the diminishing physique of our people, ascribed to their transfer from rural districts to large towns. In reference to this point I may allude to the words of Sir Thomas Crawford in his recent address at Dublin (*British Medical Journal*, August 13th, 1887): "A careful examination," he says of these tables (tables of the causes of rejection of recruits for the army), "leads to the inference that the lower classes, from whom recruits for the army are chiefly taken, are of inferior physique now to what they were twenty-five years ago." If the physique is becoming less good, must we not expect to find a proportionate diminution of the instances of great longevity ? Sir Thomas Crawford's statistics have not passed without

H. C.   8

criticism ; but, at any rate, it is a matter deserving serious attention[1].

The average WEIGHT of 227 men, in whom it is given as under 11 stone, and of 114 women as about 9 stone, is, especially in the women, small in proportion to the height and well-developed forms of these old people, and corresponds with the 'spare' condition noticed in so many, and shows that people usually become of less bodily weight as they grow older. These well-developed, and for the most part slender, figures maintain gallantly that erect attitude which is the special feature of the human form, forasmuch as we find 62 per cent. are stated to be 'erect,' and 28 per cent. only to be 'bent.'

The 'anæmic' and 'pale' condition of a large proportion

---

[1] Mr Charles Roberts, for instance (" The Physical Condition of the Masses," in the *Fortnightly Review*, October, 1887), has been led by a careful examination of the same statistics to conclusions quite opposite to those at which Sir Thomas Crawford has arrived. He finds that improvement in sanitation has not only made the population more healthy, but has materially lengthened the term of life. " Stature and weight of body," he says, " are very much matters of race, and vary in different parts of the country according to the racial origin of the inhabitants. In Scotland and the north of England the men are tall and heavy (from 5 feet 8 to 10 inches, and from 11 to 13 stone), while in the east of England they are tall but less bulky. In the southern parts of England men are much shorter and lighter of weight than in the north and east (5 feet 6 to 7 inches, and $9\frac{1}{2}$ to $10\frac{1}{2}$ stone), while in Wales they are also short, but very heavy in proportion to their stature. The adult inhabitants of towns do not fall much below that of the adjoining districts in either stature or weight. The average stature of the much-abused cockney is 5 feet 7 inches, only half an inch short of that of the whole kingdom, and higher than that of all the home counties."

(respectively 58 per cent. and 30 per cent.) accords with the fact noted in my account of the *post-mortem* examinations of centenarians (p. 103) that the spleen, lymphatic glands, and other blood-making organs are in a comparatively atrophic state in the aged. Nevertheless, it is to be remarked that a good proportion (63 per cent.) are noted to be 'strong' or of 'average' strength, as against 36 per cent., who are described as 'feeble.'

Among these old people, as in the case of the centenarians, a large number (80 per cent.) retained good SIGHT; and this evidence is confirmatory of the view, derived from the records of the centenarians, that the occurrence, even the early occurrence, of presbyopia (83 per cent. used glasses) does not militate against the continuance of good sight to a very late period of life.

It does not appear that much is to be inferred from the presence or absence of the *arcus senilis*, forasmuch as it is noted to exist in 'considerable' degree in 25 per cent., in 'slight' degree in 37 per cent., and to be 'absent' in 37 per cent.

HEARING failed in a larger proportion than sight, being reported as 'indifferent' or 'bad' in nearly half the number of returns under that head. The failure of this sense in a larger number than that of vision is probably due in great measure, as said (p. 152), to the liability of the delicate mechanism of the middle part

8—2

of the ear—the tympanum, with its bones, joints, membranes, muscles, and lining membrane—to impairment from colds, shocks, and a variety of other causes.

The good general condition, the good performance, that is, of the various functions, in a large number of these old people, is, as in the case of the centenarians, a noteworthy fact, and contributes, it need scarcely be said, in very large measure to the comfort and happiness of old age. In 71 per cent. the DIGESTION, and in 62 per cent. the APPETITE, is stated to be 'good.' In only 4 per cent. is the former, and in only 5·4 per cent. is the latter, said to be 'bad.' In 69 per cent. the bowels acted daily; and in few does it appear that they gave trouble. Very few resort to aperients; and it could be wished that a greater number of the young and middle-aged persons in the upper ranks of life would follow the example of the old people in this respect.

The process of MICTURITION is found to be natural in 83 per cent. of the women, and in 58 per cent. of the men. In 20 per cent. of the men, and in less than 3 per cent. of the women, it is noted as being slow; whereas incontinence is said to exist in about 5 per cent. of the women, and in only 3 per cent. of the men. Frequency of micturition appears to be a source of annoyance in not more than 3 per cent. or 4 per cent. in either sex.

The evidence of sound BRAIN-CONDITION is furnished

by the report of an 'average' amount of intelligence in
74 per cent.; in 15 per cent. it is stated to be 'high,' and
in 11 per cent. only to be 'low.' The memory also is in
most instances reported to be 'good,' especially (in 78
per cent.) for past events. The recent impressions, as is
the case with most of us after youth, are less durable;
still as many as 59 per cent. of these old people are
noted to have good memory for recent events. A further
evidence of good brain-condition is furnished by the observation that only 9 per cent. are bad sleepers, whereas
64 per cent. are said to be good sleepers, and 27 per
cent. to be moderately good sleepers. This does not quite
accord with what seems to be a generally received impression that the sleeping faculty of the aged is indifferent.
It may be, and it probably is, the case that the work
which should go on in sleeping, that is the repair of the
ordinary wear and tear associated with the exercise of the
various functions, and more particularly of the brain-
functions, proceeds slowly, and that a proportionately long
period is required for it; so that, although the 'sleeping
faculty' may be good, the 'sleeping power' may be less
than in earlier life. This sluggishness of the nutritive
processes in carrying on renewal after the wear attendant
upon functional exercise, and which is an appropriate
associate with the sluggishness or diminution of functional
activity in the aged, seems at first thought to be scarcely

compatible with that good performance, in these same persons, of repair after the greater lesions by wounds and ulcers to which I have before called attention. The apparent paradox, however, is probably explained, as mentioned in the report on the maladies of old people (p. 153), by the lower sensitiveness, excitability, and activity of the tissues in the aged, and by the better opportunity thus afforded for the quiet operation of the healing processes.

The disappearance of the TEETH, as remarked in former reports, does not portend so much as is commonly supposed. In 41 per cent. they were all gone, and in some this had been the case for many years. We find, moreover, in these analyses confirmation of the observations before made as a result of our investigation, that the teeth disappear at an earlier period and more commonly in women than in men, though the former are the more long-lived—the proportion in which they were absent being 52 per cent. in the women and 30 per cent. in the men— also that they disappear in the upper jaw earlier than in the lower jaw. Our reports are drawn chiefly from the class of persons who are not able to make amends for natural deficiencies by artificial aids. Thus thirty-seven only out of the whole number had artificial teeth; some of these had used them for many years. We can scarcely, therefore, draw inferences from this information respecting the advantage to health and the prolongation of life which may be afforded by the dentist's skill; although it can scarcely be doubted that benefit in these respects, as well as in comfort and other ways, will be found to result from the science and art of dentistry, which is making such great advances.

It is interesting to note that the PULSE-RATE between the ages of 80 and 100, which in the whole number of the cases observed averages 77, is about the same as that of middle-life. The slight excess above the average of middle-life may be accounted for by the presence of a certain amount of chest-affection in some of these old people. In the women the average (79) somewhat exceeds that of the men, which is 75. In 80 per cent. it is said to be regular, and in 20 per cent. to be irregular. In the greater number (60 per cent.) the pulse is described as small, and in by far the greater number (81 per cent.) as compressible. Hence the ordinary pulse of the old person may be said to be 77, regular, small, and compressible; and this may be called the 'pulse of endurance.' It indicates that the heart beats quietly and steadily, and that the arterial system is sound. In confirmation of the latter point, we find an absence of evidence of arterial disease noted in 72 per cent.; in 21 per cent. the arteries are described as being 'tortuous,' and in 12 per cent. only as being 'knotty.' I am rather surprised that the men and women are about equal in this respect, for I had supposed calcareous and other like degenerative changes in the tissues, especially in the arteries, to be more common in men than in women; and I think it would be found to be so at an earlier period of life (from sixty to eighty). In older people intemperance and other exciting causes of tissue-degeneration, which are most operative among men, have commonly been throughout life in comparative abeyance, and the natural processes have had more fair and equal play in men and in women. The importance of this will be inferred from what is said on the subject of arterial degeneration at p. 145.

The RESPIRATION, averaging about 21, is rather less frequent than might have been expected, considering the liability to bronchitis, as well as the diminishing elasticity of the pulmonary tissues and of the chest-walls, which must, to a greater or less extent, form one of the senile changes; but it accords with the observations that a comparatively good maintenance of elasticity, that is of good tissue-structure, is one of the features associated with longevity; and our tables indicate that the elasticity of the chest-wall was fairly distinguishable in about one-half of those in whom a return on this point was made. Moreover, the chest-measurement, averaging about 36 inches in inspiration and 35 in expiration in the men, and 31 in inspiration and 30 in expiration in the women, is a fair medium, and shows that, considering the time of life, the range of respiratory movement is well maintained. It is also to be noted that, in a large proportion, the voice is stated to be clear, loud and full, evidencing a sound condition, as well probably as a good development, of the vocal apparatus, a point upon which Sir Duncan Gibb is known to have laid much stress.

It is very satisfactory to find that nearly a half are reported to be of 'placid' DISPOSITION, and 45 per cent. to be still 'energetic' and brisk, whereas 17 per cent. only are said to be rather 'irritable.' With regard to several it is noted that these qualities are combined. Thus, some are stated to be 'placid' and 'energetic,' and some to be 'irritable' and 'energetic;' but, on the whole, the placid and energetic dispositions much predominate.

With regard to HABITS, 54 per cent. are stated to be 'active,' and taking more or less out-of-door exercise; 31 per cent. to be 'sedentary,' and 14 per cent. to be 'confined to bed.' Though the last is rather a large number, it must be remembered that many solaces attend upon this condition, not the least being the enjoyment of rest, which to the weary body is a real luxury. The need for it is usually, in the first instance, caused by weakness, perhaps rheumatic, in the lower limbs. These parts of the frame, which are the latest to be developed in size and strength, are the most prone to defect, disease, and debility. There is no doubt that in many cases confinement to bed leads to prolongation of life by the immunity it affords from exposures, and by its reservation to the organs essential to life of so much nerve-force and nutritive energy as is economised by the diminution of bodily activity.

The greater number (60 per cent.) are 'moderate' EATERS, 30 per cent. are 'small' eaters, and 9 per cent. only are 'large' eaters. A fair proportion (40 per cent.) are in the habit of taking a little alcohol, which, in the form of beer, whisky, or brandy, they feel to be a comfort and support, alleviating the sense of sinking which many feel; and perhaps this small quantity, especially if taken in the latter part of the day, does some real good. A smaller proportion take rather more, and are classed as 'moderate' DRINKERS. A considerable number, however, 36 per cent., take none at all, and very few (2·5 per cent.) are described as taking much. It is also observed that a large number (62 per cent.) take but little animal food; 32 per cent. partake of it moderately; 3 per cent. take none at all; and 1·1 per cent. only take it in considerable quantity. It may commonly be observed that as persons advance in years and lessen in activity, the inclination for animal food diminishes. Most of our old people are content with about three meals a day. We now and then meet with old persons who eat rather ravenously and frequently, thinking perhaps that it is necessary to do so in order to maintain their strength, and that the need for so doing is indicated by the sense of sinking at the stomach which they experience. These instances however are very exceptional; and it is probable that a small quantity of cod-liver oil, taken once or twice daily in a little wine or spirit, would relieve the sense of sinking, and would promote digestion and nutrition, and so maintain strength in a safer and better manner than an extra and quickly swallowed amount of food.

CHAPTER VII.

REPORT ON THE PAST LIFE-HISTORY OF AGED PERSONS.

THE following account of the past life-history of the 824 aged persons is a sequel to the account of their present condition, and is taken from the same analyses.

It may be remarked, in the first place, that nearly a fourth (24 per cent.) were ' first children'[1], and at least 17 of the number were 'only children,' though the greater number were about the third or fourth in the family. In 196 instances, in which the ages of the fathers and mothers at the time of the birth of the children were included in the returns, the average age of the fathers was 34, and that of the mothers 32. This would indicate the age of about 30 to be, as we might expect, so far as the offspring are concerned, the most favourable for child-producing. Five are stated to have been 'twins.' A gentleman of my acquaintance, above 80, himself a twin, married a twin, and has a large family of very healthy

[1] See remarks on this point in 'Centenarians' (p. 41).

children and several grandchildren, thus proving that the reproductive as well as the enduring qualities may be fully possessed by twins.

Of the 335 who are stated to have been MARRIED, the average age at which they were married was 29, the average duration of their married life was forty-five years, and the average number of their children was six.

Of the 292 women who are stated to have been MARRIED, the average age at which they married was 26, the average duration of their married life was forty years, and the average number of their children was six. The shorter term of married life of the women as compared with that of the men is explained by the fact that men are, on the whole, somewhat shorter-lived than women, and also that they marry at a rather later age, the term of the married life of the woman being, therefore, curtailed by the earlier deaths of the men. Not much information has been given respecting the labours of the women ; and it may, therefore, be probably inferred that they did not in most instances present any very remarkable features. One woman is stated to have had severe flooding after a confinement at the age of 42, and to have rallied with difficulty. Two had many miscarriages. In the case of one, each of her fourteen labours was by the aid of instruments, and most of the children were born dead. One had twin daughters, both of whom were alive

at the age of 56, and had large families.   Fifty-seven of
the married women were childless.   It appears, therefore,
that longevity was about equally shared by the single and
the married, by those who had borne children and those
who had not.   At the same time, among those who had
children, fertility, which imports soundness and activity
of the generative organs, is indicated to have been an
associate of longevity.

The greater proportion (55 per cent.) of these old
people had lived in comfortable circumstances, 35 per
cent. had been 'poor,' and 10 per cent. had been 'affluent.'
The greater number had been of average stoutness or of
spare habit.   Eight per cent. are said to have been 'delicate,' whereas 54 per cent. are reported to have been
'robust' throughout life, and 37 per cent. to have been
about 'average' in this respect.   Ninety per cent. had
always enjoyed good health with the exception in some,
of occasional illnesses, subsequently mentioned, which do
not appear materially to have affected their general health.
In the category of 'good health' are comprised good
digestion, which is reported with regard to 92 per cent.;
good appetite, which is noted in 88 per cent.; and good,
regular action of the bowels, which had taken place,
and in most instances daily, in 85 per cent., costiveness
being noted as habitual or frequent in only 10 per cent.

With regard to DIET we find that the smallest pro-

portion (15 per cent.) had been habitually ' large ' eaters,
20 per cent. had been 'small' eaters, and the largest
proportion (61 per cent.) had been 'average' in this respect. Five per cent. only had been in the habit of
taking 'much' animal food—that is, more than a pound
of meat daily; 38 per cent. took ' little '—that is, less than
half a pound; and 53 per cent. had been accustomed to
partake of it ' moderately '—that is, from half a pound to
a pound in the day. Fifteen per cent. had taken no
alcoholic drink at all throughout the whole or greater
part of their lives; 40 per cent. had been in the habit of
taking a 'little'—that is, less than a pint of beer or
two glasses of wine ; 33 per cent. had been accustomed to
take it in ' moderation '—that is, one or two pints of beer
daily; and less than 9 per cent. had taken more than this.
The last number is composed chiefly of men who lived to
between 80 and 90 ; with respect to the men between
these ages, of whom there were 298 returns under this
head, it is to be observed that 15 per cent. appear to have
drank rather freely—2 or more pints of beer daily—and
10 or 12 had drunk rather heavily for a portion or
throughout the greater part of their lives. These exceptional cases scarcely detract from the value of the important confirmation which our tables afford of that which
good sense suggests and which ordinary observation tells
—namely, that abstinence from, or a spare or moderate

partaking of alcoholic drinks, as well as spare or moderate eating, and spare or moderate meat-eating are most compatible with health and most conducive to the prolongation of life. In this respect the poor are at some advantage as compared with the rich, for it is quite possible—indeed, very easy—to have too much of good things in the way of food, especially when they are made agreeable to the palate; and out of the abundance of what is good much that is evil is likely to ensue. Persons are apt to forget that limitation in quantity in any article of food is one of the requisites for its wholesomeness and good nutritious effect, and that what is wholesome in moderation becomes unwholesome when the bounds of moderation are exceeded, those bounds being set by the real requirements of the system and the brisk, complete appropriative powers of the stomach and nutritive organs; and they need the caution, as I have elsewhere expressed, that "the body quickly finds for idle food some mischief sure to do."

In the able and valuable report by Dr Isambard Owen (*British Medical Journal*, June 23, 1888, p. 1312), on a "Collective Investigation Inquiry into the Connection of Disease with Habits of Intemperance," it is stated that in 4,234 returns made the average duration of life was greatest (62 years) in those who were designated "temperate"—that is, those who drink small amounts and only with meals, and rarely take spirits—and that a gradual diminution, amounting in all to rather more than ten years, was found to take place in passing down the scale to the decidedly intemperate; further, that the average duration of life reported in the case of the 'total-abstainers' was less than that reported in the 'temperate.' Some considerations, such as the preponderance of early ages among living total abstainers and the consequent greater opportunities for early death among the members of this class who were reported on in comparison with others, prevent our drawing any absolute conclusion from the last part of the statement. Still, allowance for such considerations being made, it does appear from the tables given by Dr Owen that length of life on the whole pertains to the temperate—or rather it should be said to the very temperate—as much as, perhaps even more than, to the total abstainers.

A greater number and a wider range of statistics would be needed to give trustworthy information respecting the influence of different occupations, modes of life, and places of dwelling upon the duration of life; but we find that by far the greater number (94 per cent.) of those included in our tables had been 'active' persons, and had led active lives, only 6 per cent. being described as 'sedentary.' The greater proportion (77 per cent.) of the men had been occupied much out of doors; this being the case, as might be expected, to less extent (33 per cent.) with

H. C. 9

the women. Of several it is remarked that they were good walkers, athletes, sportsmen, etc. Nothing, perhaps, more surely than good enduring power in walking, running, or similar exercise, indicates that soundness of frame and that nutritive energy and good balance of organs which lead to longevity. Moreover, the opportunity for nutrition to do its restorative work was in nearly all provided by the faculty of 'good sleeping,' to which was commonly added its appropriate attendant, the habit of 'early rising.' I say 'appropriate attendant' for 'good' sleeping is, for the most part 'quick' sleeping, that is, the reparative work which has to be done in sleep is done briskly and well. Good sleepers, in the prime of life, do not usually sleep very long, especially when they are well and actively and happily employed during the day ; and we are sometimes surprised at the small amount of sleep which those who are actively employed seem to require, the fact being that activity and energy of the will and the volitional system induce activity and energy in the sleeping or restorative operations, and, conversely, a dawdling day is commonly followed by dawdling sleep or drowsiness at night. When we speak of early rising, it must be observed that the word 'early' has a relative significance with reference to the time of going to bed. A person who retires to rest four hours after midnight and gets up at 10 A.M., may be strictly regarded as an 'early riser.'

As we found in the case of centenarians with regard to the HAIR, so in the old people we are considering it had held its ground and its colour well, the proportion of those who were bald 'early' being about 26 per cent., whereas those in whom it was noted that this had not taken place amounted to 72 per cent. Those who were grey 'early' are 24 per cent., whereas in 75 per cent. this change is said to have been 'late.'

Sixty-nine per cent. had been of 'ENERGETIC' TEMPERAMENT, giving us the satisfaction of finding energy thus associated with the qualities that promote longevity, and that good working and good wearing qualities are commonly linked together. Thirty-six per cent. are reported to have been of 'placid' temperament, and 13 per cent. to have come under the designation of 'irritable.' In a few (5 per cent.) only is the INTELLECT described as having been 'low;' in 21 per cent. it is said to have been 'high;' and 73 per cent. are said to have possessed an 'average' amount of intelligence.

It may seem somewhat remarkable that nearly one-half had suffered ILLNESSES, more or less severe, at some period or periods of life. Of these illnesses many were caused by some external influences or poisons, such as those of fever, small-pox, or scarlatina, and they therefore had no special relation to weakness, disorder, or defect in the body. Though often directly destructive of life and

9—2

seriously damaging to organs, they do not infrequently,
even when severe, pass away like a cloud and leave the
body quite unscathed, the only remaining vestige of incomplete recovery, that is, of incomplete restoration to the
previous condition, being perhaps the change, whatever it
be, which renders the system insensible to the influence
of the poison, and so confers an immunity from the recur-
rence of the particular disease. Moreover, certain local inflammatory affections, those of the lungs, for instance, and
some other parts, erysipelas, and a variety of affections,
are in like manner engendered by, or are attributable
to, poisonous or malarial agencies introduced from without, while some, of which gout may be taken as a type,
are the result of noxious materials engendered within the
body. Whatever view may be taken of the causes and
nature of the illnesses which had been undergone by
these old people—and they were of various kinds—it is
interesting to learn that in so many instances illness,
though severe, did not prevent the sufferer from reaching
old age. Doubtless the qualities which lead to old age
are those which best promote complete recovery from illness as well as complete nutritive reparation under other
circumstances; and, in relation to this subject, I may refer,
especially with regard to affections of the nervous system,
to the remarks on the Maladies of Old People (p. 147).

The minor AILMENTS with which a small proportion

had been troubled at various periods in their lives may
not have been altogether without their compensating advantages, forasmuch as these disorders not infrequently
clear away slight accumulations of evil which would otherwise have increased and festered into graver maladies.
These ailments, moreover, often serve as kindly warnings
against indiscretions and exposures which, if continued,
might prove disastrous.   Though it is better not to err at
all, it is a saving thing to be stopped or recalled in time.
Thirty-nine of the whole number (824) had suffered occasional attacks of bronchitis; 41 had been troubled with
dyspepsia; and 30 with rheumatism.   A few gave accounts of skin-eruptions—eczema or psoriasis—more or
less troublesome; others of gout, varix, or sore leg.   Still,
more than 50 per cent. appear to have passed their lives
in freedom from these and other maladies.   Our statistics, therefore, are confirmatory of the view that the
qualities which lead to old age are those which for the
most part give immunity from ailment and disease, and
which also promote recovery from them when they occur.

With regard to FAMILY HISTORY, this subject has been
so much dwelt upon and so worked out in connection
with life-insurance that little remains to be said.   In
many of our cases no sufficient information respecting it
could be obtained.   Still, 406 are reported to have be-
longed to long-lived families, those only being included

in this number in the case of whom four of the immediate
relatives (grandparents, parents, brothers or sisters) had
attained to the age of 70, or three to the age of 80. In
six instances the families are stated to have been "short-
lived." It should be added that in more than 20 per cent.
the families, on one or both sides, are stated to have been
consumptive (see also page 13), and in the families of 17
per cent. there is said to have been cancer or some form
of malignant disease.

In 367 instances, in which returns on BLOOD-RELA-
TIONSHIP are given, it is stated that none such existed
between the grandparents or between the parents in 357.
In four instances the grandparents were said to have been
cousins; and in six instances the parents are said to have
been cousins; and it is probable that in all these the relationship was that of first cousin. I do not know the proportion which the marriages of cousins bear to those in
which no such relationship exists, or what is the numerical proportion of the children of cousins to the population generally; but the fact that 10 out of 367, with
respect to whom a return on this point was made, or
rather more than 2·7 per cent., were the children of
cousins, seems to place the offspring of cousins in a very
fair position with regard to the prospects of longevity.

The results of this collective investigation respecting
aged people have not been such as to evolve anything

very novel or startling, or to give rise to any fresh theo-
ries with regard to longevity and the means of attaining
it, but rather to dissipate certain ideas which are more or
less current though founded upon too limited observation,
and to show that the maxims and laws which common
sense and sound reason would dictate hold good, that the
real *elixir vitœ* is to be found in the observance of them,
and that, as a general rule, those persons live the longest
who might be expected to do so.   Thus:—

1. The prime requisite is the faculty of age in the
blood by INHERITANCE; in other words, that the body
has been wound up, as it were, and sent into the world
with the initial force necessary to carry on the living
processes through a long period, that this is the case with
every organ, and that the several organs are so adjusted
to one another as to form a well-balanced whole.   The
various functions will then be equably and harmoniously
performed, and there will, consequently, throughout life,
be little cognisance of imperfection or ailment of any kind.

2. The body is usually WELL DEVELOPED and well
proportioned and rather spare, and, though there are many
exceptions to this, rather exceeds the average standard of
height.   It is capable of much endurance and of quick
and complete restoration after fatigue, this latter faculty
giving the habit of, and probably the desire for, early
rising; and with it also is associated a good power of

recovery from the disturbances caused by accident or disease. The cerebral or intellectual powers accord with the general good quality, and the whole nervous system is active and energetic without being irritable. The chest is broad, breadth of chest be it remarked being one of the peculiarities of the human form; it is capable of much expansion and therefore of drawing and holding a long breath. Hence the work of breathing, which has to be repeated some twenty times in a minute throughout life, takes place easily and quietly and, therefore, with comparatively little wear and tear. The heart also does its work quietly, steadily, and at moderate rate.

With regard to these points it may be observed that at birth the head is large in proportion to the rest of the body, first, because it is important for the brain to be early cased in and protected by bone, and, secondly, because when it is so cased in growth takes place with difficulty. The brain therefore in early life is large and rather soft and, as years go on, it becomes firmer but not much larger. Hence one of the factors in development after birth is to bring up the rest of the frame into due proportion to the brain and head. When this does not take place, owing either to the head being too large or to the growth of the rest of the person being insufficient, the standard of health and strength, especially in the former case, is liable to be defective. Also, when the growth of

the rest of the body is in excess, causing a disproportion
in the opposite direction, namely a lankiness of limb with
relative smallness of head, the health-standard is liable to
be low. It will commonly be found that the form of body
which to the eye gives the best proportions between head,
chest, abdomen and limbs, is the one in which the health-
standard is highest and the prospect of longevity greatest.

3. Owing to the inherent good quality of the nutritive
processes, those degenerative changes which, in advancing
years, always more or less diminish the elasticity of the
arterial coats and of other parts, are slow to occur, so that
the pulse retains, in great measure, its softness and the
thorax its vital capacity, while stiffness of limb and general
feebleness are late in their manifestation. The decadence
of the teeth, which in the animal world generally sounds
a death-knell, inasmuch as it deprives the body of the
means of obtaining its subsistence, does not seem to augur
much in the case of civilised man, to whom the teeth are
less directly needed for his maintenance; while another
cuticular appendage, the hair, seems to share, to some
extent, the enduring quality of the rest of the system.

4. To this natural long-livedness must be added the
fair opportunities for the career of the body through the
ascending and descending stages of the course assigned to
it. That course will not be exceeded, but it may be, and
usually is, curtailed. Indeed, as we know, even in those

endowed with the greatest perfection of physique, the natural life-period is, owing to a variety of circumstances more or less unfavourable and often unavoidable, rarely completed, and the normal processes of decay and dissolution are seldom allowed to have their regular course. In the domain of Nature, as I have before said, these processes are not suffered to advance very far, for the simple reason that the weakness associated with them causes the animal to fall a victim to some one of the various methods of killing which may, hence, be said to constitute the natural manner of death. Under the saving influences of civilisation, by which the rough and ready law of killing is modified, that which most contributes to the prolongation of life and the consummation of the inherited period, is "temperance in all things," especially in eating and drinking, and above all in alcoholic drinking, and to a large extent also in meat-eating. If the world did but realise, and would have the good sense and self-restraint to act upon the knowledge, that a large proportion of the ills to which man is regarded as the heir, and which are therefore looked upon as inevitable, are simply the result of excess in eating and drinking, a great addition would be made to the average term of human life and health, as well as a great economy in the consumption of the materials—the food-stuffs—by which life is sustained. This saving would probably more than compen-

sate for the additional requirement made by the addition
to life. Under the term "excesses" must especially be
included those small day-by-day superfluities which attract
little attention and are thought little of, but the in-
sinuating evil of which accumulates surely, inducing often,
in the first instance, a sense of weakness; and this is
thought to imply a need for more of that food or stimulus
which is in reality the cause of the weakness. Thus are
gradually sown the seeds of disease the true cause of
which is overlooked and which is therefore attributed to
some other cause. "Temperance" is the great lesson
under this head which our tables teach; and its importance, overshadowing as it does all others, is a reason for
not now diverting attention from it by mentioning them.

I would not restrict temperance in drinking to temperance in alcoholic drinks alone, but to the consumption
of fluids of all kinds, which should be limited to the
requirements indicated by natural thirst. By 'natural
thirst' I mean the thirst of the natural or healthy body,
which gives the true indication of the amount of fluid that
is required to maintain the softness, suppleness, and functional activity of the tissues as well as to supply the loss
by the kidneys and skin incurred in the processes of
draining away effete materials and regulating temperature.
In the ordinary working of the healthy body thirst is
slight, and healthy persons are scarcely conscious of it.

But it is liable to be increased by indulgence, and may become a dominating sensation, or an irresistible craving, in those who yield frequently to the desire to assuage it; and the passage of too much liquid through the system is injurious in a variety of ways, producing waste of material, weakening of the nutritive processes, and causing excess of wear in various organs. For this reason I have never regarded with an altogether favourable eye the 'drinking fountains' and 'temperance stalls' which well-meaning people place in our streets, having some apprehension that the facilities for drink thus afforded will promote thirst which in itself is no good omen and which probably will not always be satiated with water and other so-called 'temperance' drinks.

5. To the recovering power—the good and often the quick recovering power—of the aged after operations, fractures and other accidents, ulcers, inflammatory and other affections, manifested in many of the returns, I have already, and perhaps sufficiently, directed attention. In confirmation of these observations, many cases have been published in the Medical Journals, and others have been privately communicated to me by medical men living in various parts of the kingdom.

6. Our returns give general evidence of the comfort and happiness of old age and of quiet enjoyment of the faculties and opportunities that remain, without the pain

of remorse at those which are lost. Not unfrequently there
is much cheerfulness and merriment, and often much, even
increased, enjoyment of the beauties of nature. One
friend writes to me that this grows with him year by
year: and I have often observed that this applies rather to
limited scenery, to appreciation of the charms of a garden,
the green landscapes of England, the quiet nooks and
dells of the Lake district, such as Wordsworth in his later
time loved, rather than to the big hills and the grand
outlines which fascinate younger eyes and offer irresistible,
too often dangerous, temptations to younger limbs. The
former, especially when cheered and warmed by sunshine,
are more in harmony with the feelings of the aged, whose
thoughts, divested of the stress of life's work, are free for
their appreciation. Indeed, when the body remains sound,
and when the aspirations are, as commonly is the case,
toned into relation with its diminishing capabilities, when
the surroundings are favourable, and the mind, freed from
the struggle of the world, can enjoy calm reflection on
the past and the future, and by a genial sympathy with
others can fulfil the mission which remains to it here of
promoting peace on earth and good will among men, the
declining days are often the happiest ones of the long
life. Finally, when the developmental processes have
carried the body through the stages of its allotted span,
the gradually thinning thread of life yields without a snap,
and the aged one passes contentedly and gently away.

CHAPTER VIII.

THE MALADIES OF OLD PEOPLE.

THE following remarks, like the reports in the two preceding Chapters, are based upon the analyses derived
from the accounts of 824 persons, between eighty and a
hundred (340 men and 282 women between eighty and
ninety, and 92 men and 110 women between ninety and
a hundred).

I may first observe that, with regard to *Diseases and
Failures of Particular Organs*, the proportion of immunities
from them was in favour of the women, amounting to 55
per cent., as compared with 35 per cent. in the case of the
men. The affections of the urinary organs especially
preponderate, as we might expect, in the men. They are,
indeed, more than twice as frequent in the men than
in the women, amounting to 42 per cent., whereas in the
women they were only 20 per cent. In the women, brain-
affections are more frequent than in the men, being in
the proportion of 16 per cent. in the women to 7 per
cent. in the men. But the failures in the heart and

in the lungs are about equal in the two sexes. It is worthy of note that 85 per cent. of the whole number are reported to be free from any evidence of rheumatic affections of the hands. The hands were selected for observation because their condition is readily ascertained and because that is a fair gauge of the rest of the system.

Of the various maladies, BRONCHITIS is the dominating one, and, superadded to debility, it is oftener than any other assigned as the cause of death. It is, indeed, including the common winter-cough, a very frequent malady in this climate at all times of life. In the aged it is liable to become persistent; and a slight increase coming upon the enfeebled circulation and general weakness of the old person often produces a fatal result. The demands on the activity of the respiratory functions are, it is true, diminishing in the aged in proportion to the diminished activity of the nutritive and other processes; but the respiratory capacity, which depends much upon the elasticity of the thoracic walls and of the pulmonary tissue, is liable to diminish in still greater ratio. Hence the respiratory movements, which are in great measure (the movement of *expiration* more particularly) the resultants of elasticity, are performed incompletely and with effort, the chest as a consequence permanently maintains more and more of the expanded or *inspiratory* state, and the expulsion of mucus from the air-passages is effected with difficulty. Thus a continual source of irritation is provided, which, on slight provocation, extends into the smaller bronchial tubes, and is reluctant to quit its hold there. In a few of our old people the affection was habitual, and had been so for years. In some there had been recurrences of attacks of considerable severity, with complete recovery, at a very advanced time of life.

It will probably accord with general experience that some combination of sedative with stimulant medicines affords more relief in these cases than any other treatment.

Bronchitis being thus one of the chief enemies of aged people, it is by guarding against the exposures which induce it, by keeping indoors or even in bed in bad weather, by residence in mild climates and by various suitable precautions, that the span of life may be much prolonged. Common observation proves this in the case of those who are in comfortable circumstances; and the experience of the union-houses, where much kindly care is taken of the aged, shows it in the case of the poor.

With regard to the HEART we do not get much evidence of disease. Some irregularity or intermission of pulse was noted in about a fifth of the cases observed. In a few there were stethoscopic indications of valvular disease without any other symptoms. Whether the œdema of the legs observed in certain cases, and which we are familiar with as an occasional temporary affection in old people, is attributable to an imperfection in the heart, or to some other cause, I do not know.

A knotty condition of the ARTERIES, indicative probably of calcareous degeneration, is reported in 12 per cent.

The large proportion in which the arteries are stated to be soft and compressible, in other words to have undergone little or no change, is important in relation to the view that it is in morbid change of the arterial coats that the seeds of disease and early decay are so commonly laid. This indeed appears to constitute, in many cases, one of the earliest, the most notable, and the most important, of the senile degenerative changes, and it has been said with some truth, that a man is as old as his arteries. The thickening and loss of elasticity of the arteries, still more the atheromatous and calcareous changes in them, and the consequent interference with the blood-current through the affected vessels, necessarily lead to impaired nutritive conditions in the various tissues, with liability to atrophic, fatty, inflammatory, hæmorrhagic, cancerous, gangrenous, and other sequences, and thus constitute, directly or indirectly, the most common cause of premature death in those who have passed the middle period of life. If these changes in the arterial walls are attributable, as they are regarded by some pathologists to be, and as they in some measure probably are, to direct

contact with and irritation by morbid constituents in the
blood flowing through the vessels, this cause of senile
decay must be referred back to imperfection in the blood-
making and digestive processes,—those processes, that is
to say, which commencing in the mouth are continued
in the stomach, the intestinal canal, in the lymphatic
system and in the blood itself, and to which the salivary
glands, the pancreas and the liver, as well as the kidneys
and skin, and indeed all the secretory and excretory
organs contribute their share. Further, the practical
point is that these digestive and blood-forming imperfections are, in no small measure, engendered by our indiscretions in subjecting the organs concerned to undue trial
by the quality, and no less by the quantity, of the food
and drink with which they are expected to cope. The
confirmation of all this is found in the fact that so many
of our aged people are stated to have been moderate in
their demands on these organs and, in other words, to
have been temperate in eating and drinking, and thus to
have retained these organs, as well as the arterial system,
in a sound, healthy condition throughout their long lives.

True, as years go on, the nutritive force of all the
tissues slowly fades, and, in the normal condition, this
takes place in all alike, that is, in equal degree. But it
seems that the blood-vessels are liable to take the lead in
this failure, induced thereto probably, as just said, by

morbid states of the blood and inducing in their turn a lowered vitality, with predisposition to disease, in the parts supplied by them.

The BRAIN-AFFECTIONS, and the recoveries from them in old people, are among the most remarkable of their maladies. We are all familiar with the fact that passing attacks of unconsciousness, whether they depend upon temporary congestion or other circulatory disturbances, or upon mere suspension of cerebral activity, or other cause, are by no means uncommon, and, though sometimes very alarming, leave often no permanent diminution of mental power. The impairment or loss of motor power in some part, as a limb, is, of course, a serious addition, forasmuch as it commonly indicates a lesion or decided failure in some locality of the brain, probably of the same nature as that which we find in similar attacks in less advanced age; and a paralytic seizure not infrequently ends the long but not necessarily strange or eventful history. But we are surprised to find how even these attacks in the aged are not infrequently more or less recovered from. Thus 25 cases are given in which brain-attacks associated with paralysis, in most instances hemiplegic, and in some also with convulsions and unconsciousness, were in greater or less degree recovered from. In some the recovery was complete. One man had three attacks of paralysis, at 82, 85, and 86; and one woman, in addition to several attacks of unconsciousness, had left hemiplegia and convulsions at 78, paralysis of the left hand at 82, and severe apoplexy at 89, after which she was able to get about again, though with weakened mind and a liability to epilepsy.

While considering this point we do not forget (as mentioned at p. 20) that in the aged person the brain is gradually and progressively shrinking, and the interspace between it and the skull caused by this shrinkage is being filled by fluid-effusion in the subarachnoid or pia mater-tissue; and there may be temporary irregularities and imperfections in this compensating adjustment of pressure of fluid on the surface and of the blood circulating in the interior, which would, to some extent, account for these cerebral attacks and also for the recoveries from them. The senile alterations in the coats of the cerebral arteries must also be an important item; but our knowledge of the physiology of the cerebral circulation is at present scarcely sufficient to enable us to make clear deductions respecting its pathology.

In only 11 out of the 340 returns of men between 80 and 90, and in only 1 of the 92 returns between 90 and 100, is PROSTATIC DISEASE said to have existed. In one of these it had existed several years, and in others two, three, and four years respectively. In one the affection is said to have given less trouble than formerly. The condition of retention relieved by frequent use of the catheter may be extended with care over many years; but the enlargement of the prostate, with its associated bladder-symptoms, is, I fear, a malady from which recovery, even in old age, is scarcely to be expected. It is something to find that our reports confirm the view (p. 25) that it is a malady from which age gives, after 70, a gradually-increasing exemption.

The enlargement of the prostate gland is apparently the result of a degenerative change, resembling the senile thickening of the arterial coats, consisting, that is to say, like it in a substitution of a continuous increment of a low fibroid tissue in place of the natural structures and occurring in this instance in and about the walls of the ducts, while the calibre of the ducts, like that of the arteries, becomes increased and their terminal parts, or acini, become dilated and sacciform. What may be the real relation, as cause or effect, between the two phenomena—the thickening of the duct-walls and the enlargement of the duct-calibre—is not easy to say. The change further resembles that in the arteries and probably also other degenerative changes, such as calcification of the costal cartilages, with respect to the period of life at which it most commonly takes place, viz. about 60, the liability diminishing after 70. Again, as in the case of the arteries, the ill effects of the change are chiefly manifested, not so much in the part primarily affected, as in parts somewhat distant and dependent on or associated with it. Thus the enlargement of the prostate may go on long and to considerable extent without deleterious consequences, provided the bladder and kidneys are not injuriously influenced by it.

Fifty-two were troubled with RHEUMATISM in some of its many forms, which include pains in the limbs, aching in the bones, etc., for which, I suppose, a remedy is not very easily to be found. Indeed, it is difficult to define precisely, or clearly account for, the various pains, rheumatic and other, which old people often complain of, and which disturb their comfort without materially affecting their health. The women suffer from these even more than the men, probably in consequence of the nervous system in them being more on the alert. These various pains are included here under the head of 'rheumatism' because they are so described, the word covering as we know a multitude of pains, rather than because they are rightly so classified. Probably the term "senile pains" would be more appropriate. They, as well as the stiffness of joints associated with old age, are not unlikely due to the deficiency of moisture and consequent want of suppleness in the joints and various tissues. Possibly also there may be some degenerative changes in the nerves. Five of the men and six of the women had GOUT, all these being between 80 and 90.

Two cases of SENILE GANGRENE were noted. They were in men above 90.

The severe forms of MALIGNANT DISEASE are not frequent. One man, above 80, had rapidly advancing sarcoma of the shoulder; 5 women, between 80 and 90, had cancer of the breast; 5 men and 1 woman had epithelioma; and 1 man and 1 woman had rodent ulcer. None of these maladies are mentioned in the men or women above 90. Still, although the very aged appear to be less liable to some of the more severe diseases, such as cancers and diseases of the urinary organs, they are, on the whole, rather more liable to a variety of ordinary and slight maladies, the proportion of those above 90 who were altogether exempt from malady being 34 per cent., while the proportion of those between 80 and 90 was 43 per cent.

With regard to the EYES, 8 per cent. are stated to suffer from cataract, 80 per cent. are said to have good sight, although 83 per cent. use glasses. Some have used glasses for many years, which is confirmatory of what I said in the account of the centenarians (p. 45), that "the occurrence of presbyopia does not seem to be associated with, or to be a prelude to, inconvenience or impairment of sight beyond that which may be corrected by glasses."

The more frequent failure of the organ of HEARING,

which is noted in more than one-half (56 per cent.) of the returns, is probably due in great measure to the liability to impairment of the delicate mechanism of the middle ear—the tympanum with its membrana tympani, its ossicles with their joints, its muscles, its Eustachian tube, and its lining membrane—in consequence of colds, shocks, and a variety of causes. But in comparing the organ of hearing with that of sight, in this respect, we must not forget that the lessening of elasticity and muscular activity—which we must assume to induce defects in hearing in old persons corresponding with the visual defects classed under the term presbyopia—does not, like the latter, admit of alleviation by an easily applied physical apparatus. At least, nothing corresponding to the portable and convenient lenses for presbyopia has yet been adapted to meet the auditory defects which may be attributed to a presbyotic condition. This doubtless causes the instances of notable deafness to be out of due proportion to those of notable deficiency in vision. To make a fairer estimate between the two conditions we should compare the instances in which slight deafness occurs with those in which glasses are required.

In 4 per cent. only is the DIGESTION said to have been bad. In 71 per cent. it is reported as good, and in the remainder moderate. Very few were troubled with constipation. In 62 per cent. the appetite is reported to be good; and by far the greater number are stated to be good sleepers.

I am continually seeing and hearing of instances confirmatory of the inference as to the good REPARATIVE POWERS of the aged after fractures, wounds, and ulcers, which were based upon the returns furnished in reply to Collective Investigation inquiries, and which I have already published[1]. These inferences are so contrary to preconceived notions, indeed, to probabilities, that it takes some time and effort and frequent repetition to obtain for them a fair measure of acceptance; but I think the reparative powers of age are becoming more accredited, and that we shall ere long cease to have age adduced as a reason against the hopeful, and therefore careful, treatment of fractures, wounds, and sores in the octogenarian, the nonagenarian, and even in the centenarian.

What is still more remarkable than the healing powers of the aged after local lesions is the reparative powers often evinced by them after illnesses, as shown by numerous examples of those between 80 and 100, and also by some of the centenarians, which have been already given (page 50). Indeed, the recoveries from severe attacks of bronchitis, pneumonia, apoplexy, and paralysis, indicate the reparative powers after illness as well as

[1] *British Medical Journal* of July 12th, 1884.

after accident to be among the most interesting of the
senile features. It is certainly strange that, when the
other nutritive forces are failing—wearing out, as it were
—those which are concerned in the work of repair, which
may be regarded as, next to development, the highest
effort of nutrition, should hold their ground so well. I
have already instanced some other conditions in which the
same contrast is observed, notably that of the healing of
the stump after separation of a part following gangræna
senilis, where the structures next to those which were
unable to maintain their vitality at all often evince so
much granulating and cicatrising energy. As an illus-
tration of this, I have at the present time, in Addenbrooke's Hospital, a man, aged 77, with calcified arteries,
in whom the right great toe and the left second toe
have mortified and separated, and the parts left have
healed well and soundly, the head of the metatarsal bone
of the hallux being covered by a large cicatrix, which
must have formed with difficulty at any period of life;
and cicatrisation is now going on rapidly on the surface
left by sloughing and ulceration on the inner side of
the left great toe. Attention has quite recently been
drawn by Dr Harley (see *Lancet* of June 18th) to certain
facts which seem to have a bearing upon this point. He
observes that high breeding in most animals conduces to a
marked diminution in the bodily recuperative capacity;

also that the higher bodily recuperative capacity shown to be possessed by all men living in a rude state, whether as savages or gipsies or tramp-wanderers among ourselves, arises from the fact that the refining influences of civilisation materially diminish the animal recuperative capacity.

We are familiar also with the great reparative powers exhibited in some of the lower animal forms as compared with those in the higher animals. It would seem that the greater sensitiveness—that is, irritability or susceptibility of the nervous system and of the tissues generally— which is associated with higher organisation, where we may suppose the balances of nutrition to be most delicately swung, are, in a measure, unfavourable to reparative work. We can quite conceive that the calm, quiet processes upon which it depends are less likely to proceed in an orderly and uninterrupted manner under conditions of high excitability, where stimulus easily engenders disorder, as in infants or children, than under lower vitality and less susceptible circumstances. Herein, possibly—namely, in the lower and slower excitability of their tissues—may be found an explanation of those recuperative powers of the aged to which I have referred, and of which it is practically important that we should take due account.

I cannot close this record without bearing testimony

to the comfort and kindness which the old people receive in the various union-houses that I have visited. They are well fed, kept warm and free from exposures, walk out when they can, and lie in bed when it suits them to do so; and great attention is paid to their cleanliness. It was obvious that mutual attachment had grown up, in most instances, between them and the master and mistress of the house and the medical and other attendants. It would, I think, tend to soothe the feelings of the unwilling ratepayer if he occasionally visited the poor-house and witnessed the comfort which the aged and infirm are deriving from that largest charity ever known—the English poor-law system—to which he, perhaps unwillingly, contributes.

CHAPTER IX.

ANALYSES OF RETURNS RESPECTING THE PRESENT CONDITION AND PAST HISTORY OF PERSONS BETWEEN EIGHTY AND A HUNDRED YEARS OLD.

FOR the following analyses of the returns respecting the present condition, including the habits and circumstances, also respecting the past history, including the family history, of 824 persons between the ages of 80 and 100, I am indebted to A. Francis, M.R.C.S., who also assisted me in making the tables from which the analyses were worked out.

Of these persons, 340 were males and 282 were females, between the ages of 80 and 90; and 92 were males and 110 were females between the ages of 90 and 100.

The analyses are derived from the Reports sent, chiefly by medical men, in reply to the inquiries of, and upon the forms issued by, the Collective Investigation Committee of the British Medical Association.

The analyses of their *Present Condition* and of their *Past Life-History* are given separately; and, for purposes of comparison, the analyses of the returns of the *Men* and *Women* are given separately, and each is given respectively in the decades from *eighty* to *ninety* and from *ninety* to a *hundred*. The analyses of the returns of persons over a hundred (the *Centenarians*) were given at a preceding page.

NO. I.

ANALYSIS OF RETURNS RELATING TO PRESENT CONDITION, HABITS, CIRCUMSTANCES, ETC.

Of MALES, from 80 to 90.

340 Returns.

SINGLE : MARRIED : WIDOWED.—335 returns; S. 36, M. 80, W. 219.

AFFLUENT : COMFORTABLE : POOR.—337 returns; A. 40, C. 138, P. 159.

FAT : SPARE : AVERAGE.—333 returns; F. 37, Sp. 114, A. 182.

FULL-BLOODED : PALE : AVERAGE.—321 returns; F. 54, P. 57, A. 210.

STRONG : FEEBLE : AVERAGE.—329 returns ; S. 106, F. 100, A. 123.

HEIGHT.—313 returns; average, a little over 5 feet 7 inches.

WEIGHT.—188 returns ; average, a little over 11 stone.

FIGURE.—299 returns ; erect 198, bent 101.

VOICE.—325 returns. Weak, 31 ; loud 57 ; clear, 81 ; full, 16 ; loud and clear, 77 ; clear and full, 44 ; clear and weak, 11 ; loud and full, 7 ; loud, clear, and full, 1.

SIGHT.—267 returns; good, 224; cataracts (both sides), 19 ; cataract (one side), 3 ; failure of sight, apparently independent of presbyopia, 21; one of them had been "blind for ten years," and one had had "opaque corneæ for twenty years."

GLASSES.—259 returns ; none, 42 ; one of these used them formerly ; 217 used glasses. In some of them the number of years during which glasses had been used was given : "All life," 3; "many years," 17; "occasionally," 1; "for small print," 1; "not long," 1; "none till 80," 1; 1 year or less, 3; 2 to 3 years, 11; 4 to 5 years, 13; 6 to 7 years, 10; 8 to 10 years, 20; 12 to 15 years, 20; 16 to 20 years, 39; 21 to 25 years, 6; 26 to 30 years, 23; 31 to 35 years, 4; 36 to 40 years, 19; 41 to 45 years, 4; 46 to 50 years, 7; 62 years, 1; 65 years, 1.

HEARING.—329 returns; good, 188; indifferent, 98; bad, 43.

JOINTS OF HAND.—330 returns; natural, 287; stiff, 17; deformed,15; stiff and deformed, 9; Dupuytren's contraction, 2.

DIGESTION.—337 returns; good, 253; moderate, 72; bad, 12.

APPETITE.—335 returns; good, 224; moderate, 95; bad, 16.

EATER.—320 returns; large, 24; moderate, 211; small, 85.

NUMBER OF MEALS.—275 returns; average rather over three daily.

ALCOHOL.—320 returns; none, 120; little, 120; moderate, 67; much, 13.

ANIMAL FOOD.—304 returns; none, 9; little, 182; moderate, 109; much, 4.

BOWELS.—313 returns; daily, 219; alternately, 23; irregular, 68; relaxed, 1; costive, 1; 3 to 4 times daily, 1.

APERIENTS.—294 returns; never, 85; occasionally, 1; rarely, 149; frequently, 59.

DISPOSITION.—328 returns; placid, 140; irritable, 33; lethargic, 7; energetic, 100; placid and lethargic, 6; placid and energetic, 25; irritable and energetic, 17.

INTELLECT.—322 returns; high, 55; average, 242; low, 25.

MEMORY.—*Past Events.*—307 returns; good, 253; moderate, 34; bad, 20. *Recent Events.*—260 returns; good, 166; moderate, 56; bad, 38.

HABITS.—327 returns; active, 202; sedentary, 93; one of these "could work, but for deafness;" bedridden, 32; of these, one for 5 weeks, two for 6 months, one for 5 years.

OUT-OF-DOOR EXERCISE.—306 returns; none, 45 (including 32 who were bedridden); little, 81; moderate, 65; of these one works still; short walks, 44; much, 71; of these one "in river daily," "two still work," one "worked until stopped by an accident 4 months ago," one "gardens," one "walks much," three "walk 3 miles," one "walks for 2 hours," one "walks and rides," two "walk 8 to 10 miles," one "walks 12 miles a day," two "hunt," one of them twice a week.

SLEEP.—326 returns; good, 230; moderate, 78; bad, 18. *Number of Hours.*—213 returns; average, $7\frac{2}{3}$ hours. *Hour of Going to Bed.*—275 returns; average, about 9 o'clock. *Hour of Rising.*—271 returns; average, about 7.10 A.M.

CHEST-GIRTH IN INSPIRATION.—167 returns; average, little over 36 inches.

CHEST-GIRTH IN EXPIRATION.—167 returns; average, little over 35 inches. Only those cases are here included in which the chest-girth both in expiration and in inspiration were returned.

ELASTICITY OF RIB CARTILAGES.—209 returns; distinct, 106; indistinct, 103.

PULSE.—280 returns; average, about 74 per minute. This average is rather high, owing to the frequent occurrence of chest-affections; a large number had pulse-rate below 70 per minute. *Regular, Irregular.*—262 returns; R. 201, I. 61. *Large, Small.*—237 returns; L. 111, S. 126. *Compressible, Incompressible.*—261 returns; C. 208, I. 53.

ARTERIES.—252 returns; even, 144; visible, 7; tortuous, 19; tortuous and even, 9; tortuous and visible, 20; visible and even, 22; tortuous, visible, and even, 2; knotty, 12; visible and knotty, 6; tortuous and knotty, 7; tortuous, visible, and knotty, 4. So that they were *even* in 177 cases, *knotty* in 29 cases, *visible* in 61 cases, *tortuous* in 61 cases.

RESPIRATION.—Number, 237 returns. Average, 20 to 21 per minute. The average is high, owing to the frequent occurrence of chest affections. *Regular, Irregular.*—252 returns. R. 242, I. 10.

ARCUS SENILIS.—266 returns. Absent, 94; little, 98; much, 74; one of these had had arcus senilis since 44 years of age.

TEETH.—300 returns; average about 6 each; but 87 had no teeth, and one of these not for 20 years. In 282 cases the teeth were specified. Upper incisors, 235; canines, 147; molars, 249; lower incisors, 438; canines, 221; molars, 330.

ARTIFICIAL TEETH.—195 returns. 158 did not use them, and of these 46 had not any teeth, and one had not had any teeth for 20 years, another not for 30 years; besides these 46 cases, many others had very few teeth. 37 used artificial teeth; for many years, 3; 35 years, 1; 32 years, 1; 30 years, 2; 28 years, 1; 20 years, 10; 17 years, 1; 15 years, 4; 12 years, 1; 10 years, 5; 9 years, 1; 6 years, 2; 4 years, 2; "yes," 3.

EVIDENCES OF FAILURE.—285 returns. None, 102; heart, 16; heart and lungs, 5; heart, lungs and brain, 1; heart, lungs, and urinary organs, 4; heart, brain, and urinary organs, 1; heart and urinary organs, 12; heart, lungs, brain, and urinary organs, 3; lungs, 29; lungs and brain, 2; lungs and urinary organs, 18; brain, 11; brain and urinary organs, 7; urinary organs, 74. In 22 cases the heart-sounds are returned as "normal."

So that the *heart* was affected in 42 cases, the *lungs* in 62

H. C.   11

cases, the *brain* in 25 cases, the *urinary organs* in 119 cases.
In the case of the urinary organs the failure was in many cases
very slight, not affecting the general health (*vide* Micturition).

MICTURITION.—267 returns.   Natural, 157 ; frequent, 14;
1 occasionally ; slow, 56 : incontinence, 7 ; one of these "for
years," one for 3 months, and one "nocturnal;" quick, 1 ;
difficult, 2 ; slow and difficult, 11, one of them "for 30 years,"
another used a catheter twice daily ; difficult and painful, 1 ;
frequent and painful, 2 ; slow and frequent, 6 ; frequent and
incontinence, 1 ; slow and painful, 2 ; slow, difficult and painful, 2 ; catheterised, 6, of these, one twice daily, one 4 times
daily, one 6 times daily, one for 3 years, one daily for 40 years
(*vide* Present Maladies).

PRESENT MALADIES.—The returns are very incomplete ; in
many cases only symptoms have been returned, in· others
failure of some organ was returned, but the nature of the
failure was not stated ; in hardly any cases have details of the
malady been given; the maladies have therefore been grouped
in relation to the organ which appeared most affected.

278 returns ; none 89.

Bronchitis. — 43 cases ; 1 frequently, 1 occasionally ; 9
chronic, and one of these for 2 years.   *Asthma.*—3 cases ;
1 chronic.   *Cough.*—5 cases.   *Dyspnœa.*—4 cases.   *Emphysema.*—8 cases ; one for 2 years.   *Congestion of Lungs.*—
3 cases ; 1 died.   *Pneumonia.*—1 case ; died.   *Chronic Naso-
pharyngeal Catarrh.*—1 case.

Debility.—24 cases ; one for 6 months.   *Weak Heart.*—
12 cases, 1 with giddiness and fainting.   *Syncope.*—1 case,
occasionally.   *Vertigo.*—1 case.   *Palpitations.*—2 cases ; one
occasional and severe for 20 years.   *Dilated R, Heart.*—1 case.

Murmurs.—7 cases; one for 2 years; systolic at base in 2, mitral in 2 (in one of these for 10 years), mitral systolic in 1, aortic in 1. *Intermittent Heart.*—2 cases; in 1 every fourth beat, in the other occasionally. *Anæmia.*—1 case, for a year.

Dyspepsia.—5 cases. *Diarrhœa.*—6 cases; two occasionally, one for 3 months, one for 16 years, one for 4 days, with death. *Piles.*—2 cases. *Fistula.*—one case for 30 years. *Prolapsus Ani.*—2 cases; one for 15 years. *Enlarged Liver.*—1 case. *Hernia.*—8 cases; 1 double, one for 10 years, one for 55 years. *Inguinal Hernia.*—15 cases; 1 double, 1 large, one large for 12 years, one large for 30 years, one for 50 years, one for 60 years. *Umbilical Hernia.*—1 case. *Headaches.*—1 case.

Enlarged Prostate.—11 cases; 1 for several years, three for 2, 3, and 4 years respectively, and one gives less trouble now than formerly. *Cystitis.*—2 cases; 1 died. *Pus in Urine.* —1 case. *Irritable Bladder.*—4 cases; one for 18 months, 1 for a few years. *Atony of Bladder.*—2 cases. *Gravel.* 1 case. *Hæmaturia.*—3 cases; 1 occasionally prostatic, 1 three attacks in last 6 months. *Retention.*—2 cases; 1 occasionally, 1 with death.

Rheumatism.—19 cases; one for 12 months, one of hip for 4 years. *Sciatica.*—4 cases. *Lumbago.*—1 case. *Gout.*— 7 cases; 1 of them in foot. *Pains in Bones.*—1 case. *Lame.*— 1 case.

Paralysis Agitans.—3 cases. *Delusions.*—1 case. *Mental Depression.*—1 case. *Insane.*—1 case for 60 years. *Epileptic Fits.*—1 case recently, 1 fit every 2 months. *Occasional Fits.* —1 case from "brain congestion." *Cerebral Hæmorrhage.*—4 cases, all died; one was the "third attack at 86." *Partial Hemiplegia.*—2 cases, one for 13 months, one for 4 years. *Paralysis of Face and Voice.*—1 case for 6 months.

11—2

Epithelioma.—5 cases; three of lip; in one of these re-moved at 84, wound healed by first intention; one of finger, removed; one of penis and prepuce, operated on two months ago. *Rodent Cancer.*—1 case, of ear. *Nasal Polypi.*—1 case. *Fibrous Tumour.*—1 case, size of hen's egg, over orbit, removed at 81 after 3 years' duration. *Sarcoma.*—1 case of shoulder, 15 months' duration, increasing rapidly, with little effect on general health.

Œdema of Legs.—5 cases, one for 14 weeks. *Enlarged Legs.*—1 case, hard and brawny. *Inflamed Legs.*—1 case. *Sore Leg.*—1 case. *Varicose Ulcers.*—4 cases; one for 6 months, one for 2 years, one for 20 years, now healing; one for 6 years. *Eczema.*—4 cases; one of ankle, one for 5 years. *Psoriasis.*—1 case. *Lupus.*—1 case, from stroke of whip. *Bedsores.*—1 case. *Senile Gangrene.*—4 cases, one of these of toe. *Ophthalmia.*—2 cases.

Erysipelas.—1 case with death. One died after "4 days' feverish illness."

Fracture of Femur.—2 cases, one "impacted, one month ago."

ANALYSIS OF RETURNS RELATING TO PAST HISTORY, INCLUDING FAMILY HISTORY.

Of MALES, from 80 to 90.

340 Returns.

Age when Married.—273 returns. Average a little over 28 years of age.

Duration of Married Life.—260 returns. Average about 43½ years.

Number of Children.—269 returns; average about 6 each, but 34 had no children.

Affluent, Comfortable, Poor.—326 returns; A. 33, C. 190, P. 103.

First, or —— Child of Parents.—303 returns; average 3rd to 4th child. In 50 cases the number in the family was also given; in these the average position was 2nd to 3rd child, and the average number in the family was 6 to 7 children; 72 were "1st child," and of these 10 at least were "only child;" one was a twin, his twin sister dying at the age of 6 months; another had twins, who were both alive at 56 years of age.

Fat, Spare, Average.—317 returns; F. 69, Sp. 100; average, 148.

Delicate, Robust, Average.—311 returns; D. 12, R. 189, A. 110.

Health, Good, Moderate.—315 returns; G. 304, M. 11.
Often, Rarely, Ailing.—14 returns; O. 7, R. 7.

Digestion.—325 returns; good, 307; indifferent, 17; bad, 1.

Bowels.—307 returns; good (daily), 266; irregular, 12; costive, 25; relaxed, 4.

Baldness.—191 returns; early, 55; late, 135; not bald, 1.

Greyness.—248 returns; early, 58; late, 189; not grey, 1.

Disposition.—308 returns; placid, 98; irritable, 19; lethargic, 2; energetic, 133; placid and energetic, 35; placid and lethargic, 2; irritable and energetic, 19.

Intellect.—308 returns; high, 68; low, 16; average, 224.

Habits.—308 returns; active, 293; sedentary, 15.

Out-of-Door Exercise.—298 returns; little, 31; (of these one "could walk 50 miles," and one "always worked indoors"); moderate, 39; one of these travelled much in Germany and America; much, 228; of these 13 were great walkers, 1 walked 20 to 30 miles a day, one " 30 miles on 4 days a week," one 5 to 20 miles daily, one " 50 miles, many a day ;" two 10 miles daily. Besides these, six had much walking, riding, or driving, or worked hard; one was an "athlete, walked 20 miles;" one "great athlete, runner, and jumper;" two were pugilists; one " active in boyish and manly exercises ;" one "much hunting;" one "hunting since 8 years old ;" one "hunting and shooting all his life;" one "hunting, drinking, shooting, fishing;" one "in saddle as doctor for 50 years ;" one " led an irregular gipsy life ;" one was at sea; one " much exposed in India for over 25 years ;" one was " engaged in whaling, and in India, leading an adventurous life."

HOURS IN BED.—243 returns. *Average.*—Nearly 8 hours.

Hours of Rising.—253 returns. *Average.*—A little before 6 A.M.

Sleeper.—311 returns. Good, 278 ; average, 26 ; bad, 7.

Appetite.—295 returns. Good, 289 ; indifferent, 6.

Eater.—305 returns. Large, 52 ; average, 194; small, 59.

Alcohol.—298 returns. *None.*—28 ; besides these, one "never till 30," and another "none after 60." *Little.*—(under 1 pint) 95 ; of these, one took a quarter and one half a pint of beer daily. *Moderate* (1 to 2 pints).—112; of these, six took 1 to 2 pints of beer or porter daily, one 4 glasses of wine, one half a pint of claret, one was an abstainer till 40, one "little in early life," one "much in early life," one took a little rum, one had "tendency to drink," one "much at times," one "did not take alcohol daily, but occasionally to excess; 4 pints of beer made him tipsy." *Much* (more than 2 pints).—45 ; of these, two were "free livers," two "much beer, free livers," one "very much beer," one "much beer regularly," two 2 to 3 pints of beer, one "2 to 4 pints of beer all his life," one 4 pints of beer daily, one 6 pints of beer often, three 3 to 5 pints of beer, one "in early life, never intemperate," one "drank heavily in early life," one "heavy drinker, able to stand large quantities," one "much of all kinds," one "much port," one "three-fourths of a bottle of Marsala for years," one "often drunk," one "freely never too much," one took 5 ounces of rum daily, one "a pint and a half of wine and spirits daily for years," one "three glasses of whisky and wine," one "6 ounces of whisky," one "drank all he could get," three "much when they could get it," one was a publican, one "drank freely of rum (1 pint daily) till 46, none since," one "took 6 pints of beer and much spirits, was a great drinker till 6 years ago, never went to bed sober if he

could get beer," one "often drank a bottle of rum before
breakfast when in Australia."

ANIMAL FOOD.—272 returns. *None.*—1. *Little* (under
half a pound).—107 ; one of these was "almost a vegetarian."
Moderate (half a pound to a pound).—143. *Much* (more than
1 pound).—21.

ILLNESSES UNDERGONE.—"*Fever.*"[1]—16 cases; one "young,"
one "40 years ago, severe," one "a year ago," and nine at
16, 20, 25, 34, 35, 40, 40, 50, and 74 respectively. *Typhus
Fever.*—16 cases ; one severe, one in childhood, and eight at
14, 20, 24, 25, 37, 40, 45, and 46 respectively, one in 1827,
one at 40, severe, two 40 and 50 years ago respectively.
Typhoid Fever.—8 cases ; two severe at 27 and 67 respectively,
five at 15, 40, 50, 55, and 60 respectively. *Yellow Fever.*—
1 case, twice. *Scarlet Fever.*—6 cases; one "young," four at
18, 40, and 40, severe, and 65, severe. *Influenza.*—1 case,
at 50. *Whooping-cough.*—1 case, at 56. *Small-pox.*—9 cases ;
one in childhood, one slightly, one at 16, severe, one at 74, one
"confluent at 19," one 77 years ago, one twice, one "in 1825
after vaccinia." *African Fever.*—1 case.

Ague.—5 cases; one "prolonged" at 20, three at 40, 44,
and 68.

Intermittent Fever.—1 case. *Erysipelas.*—5 cases ; one
" of leg often," one at 81 recovered, one severe 50 years ago.
Cellulitis.—2 cases ; one at 82 with incisions, one three times
at 65, 75, and 80.

Cholera.—3 cases, one at 30. *Dysentery.*—2 cases, one at
82, one in 1883. *Syphilis.*—1 case. *Carbuncle.*—5 cases, one
had two, one 20 years ago, three at 60, 74, and 75, the last
with incisions and quick recovery.

[1] Probably many of the cases designated "*Fever*" and "*Typhus
Fever*" were "*Typhoid Fever.*"

Brain Fever.—2 cases at 30 and 46. *Sunstroke.*—1 case at 50. *Adder Bite.*—1 case.

"*Cerebral Affection.*"—1 case, 30 years ago. *Rheumatic Fever.*—14 cases, two "young," two 30 and 40 years ago, nine at 20, 34, 40 (severe), 42 (severe, with complete recovery), 45, 58, 60, 63, and 65. *Chorea.*—1 case. *Rheumatism.*—6 cases, one twice, one 12 years ago, one for 12 years. *Rheumatic Gout.*—1 case at 37. *Gout.*—10 cases, one occasionally, one frequently, one frequently for 10 years, one for 17 years, one since 21 years old, with chalk stones in fingers. *Sciatica.*—3 cases, one at 69. *Lumbago.*—1 case. *Neuralgia.*—3 cases; one at 55, one in legs with insomnia at 55 and with issues for 8 years.—*Rheumatic Iritis.*—1 case, 25 years ago. *Lithotomy.*—1 case, 15 years ago, removal of large uric acid calculus. *Lithotrity.*—1 case, 24 years ago. *Lithuria.*—1 case. *Renal Colic.*—1 case, 50 years ago.

Hæmatemesis.—1 case. *Jaundice.*—3 cases; one at 84 severe, one at 81 recovered. *Gall-stones.*—4 cases; one for 34 years. *Hepatic Abscess.*—1 case bursting into colon at 43. *Hepatitis.*—2 cases, in one two attacks at 30 and 35. *Bilious Attacks.*—1 case occasionally. *Hepatic Congestion.*—1 case occasionally. *Colic.*—2 cases; one severe a year ago. *Dropsy.*—1 case, 5 years ago, tapped 6 quarts, recovered. *Diarrhœa.*—1 case at 85. *Typhlitis.*—1 case at 40. *Inflammation of Bowels.*—2 cases, one at 21.

Hæmaturia.—1 case, 3 attacks in 6 months. *Albuminuria.*—2 cases; one 4 years ago, one 1 year ago for a few days. *Irritable Bladder.*—2 cases; one a few years ago, one from 50 to 60. *Retention.*—1 case, catheterised twice daily for one month, with recovery. *Difficult Micturition.*—1 case at 68, catheterised then and occasionally since. *Disease of*

Bladder and Prostate.—1 case, severe, from 72 to 78, now quite well. *Stricture.*—1 case when young.

Diseased Hip.—1 case in infancy, lame. *Syncope.*—1 case at 74. *Bled.*—2 cases; one for illness at 40, one for transfusion. *Epistaxis.*—2 cases; severe at 30 and 73; one was thought to be dying 15 years ago. *Fistula.*—1 case 50 years ago. *Sarcoma of Eye.*—1 case. *Abscess.*—4 cases; one of thigh 50 years ago, one "strumous when young;" one of "shoulder at 76, recovery;" one in "side at 30, in bed 8 weeks."

Bronchitis.—23 cases; one "severe," three "severe" at 47, 60, and 84; two at 65 and 68; four 6 months, 6 months, 10 years, and 17 years ago; one "several attacks since 80;" one "3 attacks severe, with recovery at 50, 83, and 84;" one "5 acute attacks in successive winters from 77 to 82 years;" one "two attacks at 50 and 75;" one "several severe attacks;" one "severe 2 years ago, recovery." *Broncho-pneumonia.*— 1 case at 82, recovery. *Œdema of Lungs.*—1 case. *Asthma.*— 1 case for 10 years. *Pulmonary Congestion.*—2 cases, at 30 and in 1875 respectively. *Bronchitis and Pleuro-pneumonia.*—1 case, three times in last 7 years, last at 84, good recovery. *Pneumonia.*—4 cases, one "two attacks at 45 and 50," one severe 10 years ago, two at 66 and 79. *Pneumonia and Pleurisy.*—1 case at 78. *Pleurisy.*—6 cases; five at 16, severe, 28, 60, 72, 82 respectively. *Phthisis.*—3 cases; two had "slight symptoms when young;" a third had "hæmoptysis at 40, in bed 8 weeks;" one was "delicate in early life;" one had "breakdown from anxiety, with diplopia and intermittent pulse at 64, with recovery;" one had "irregular heart 10 years ago, from study; recovering with change."

Epilepsy.—2 cases; one 20 to 30, fits in last two years,

failure of memory. *Insane.*—1 case. *Apoplexy and Paralysis.*—
16 cases; one "20 years ago, partial paralysis of right arm
for 5 years, recovery;" one "in 1850, with right hemiplegia;"
one "convulsions on right side with unconsciousness, a year
ago with recovery;" one "fit at 79, with hemiplegia, complete
recovery except of voice;" one "hemiplegia a year ago," one
"left hemiplegia at 76," one "3 attacks at 82, 85, and 86;"
one "paralysis at 65;" one "slight stroke at 85, slight
paralysis after;" one "slight stroke lately, weak after;" one
"paralysis of both legs and left arm, not unconscious, quite
recovered;" one "paralysis at 84, partial recovery, died of
apoplexy;" one "hemiplegia at 45, recovery;" one "hemiplegia
at 84, nearly recovered;" one "right hemiplegia and aphonia
at 84, recovered." *Congestion of Brain.*—1 case at 62.

SLIGHT AILMENTS.—256 returns; none, 156. One was
"ailing till 50," one had "feeble childhood and youth, health
and appetite better after 80."

Bronchitis.—16 cases; one "several times," four chronic.
Cough.—2 cases; one frequently. *Catarrh.*—1 case. *Asthma.*—
1 case, 28 years.

Dyspepsia.—16 cases; one lately, one at 70, recovery.
Bilious Attacks.—3 cases. *Giddiness.*—2 cases; one occasionally, one "after meals." *Flatulence.*—1 case. *Gall-stones.*—
1 case. *Palpitations.*—3 cases; one occasionally, one "for 20
years."

Headaches.—3 cases; of these one "sick headaches every 3
months," one "sick headaches frequently." *Constipation.*—4
cases.

Diarrhœa.—8 cases; one "in summer," two occasionally, one
has "tendency to diarrhœa," one "for 15 years, since injury
to abdomen." *Piles.*—3 cases. *Epistaxis.*—1 case.

Rheumatism.—16 cases; one at 68, one "lately, in bed 3 months." *Gout.*—7 cases; one slight, one annually for 30 years, two occasionally. *Sciatica.*—2 cases. *Neuralgia.*—1 case. *Angina.*—1 case rarely.

Ague.—1 case. *Orchitis.*—1 case occasionally. *Hernia.*— 6 cases; one double, one "from infancy," one for 30 years, one "inguinal," one "right inguinal," and one "inguinal for 30 years."

Difficult Micturition.—1 case, few years ago, from stricture.

Eczema.—7 cases; one "of legs," one at 46, one "30 years of leg," two for 2 and 4 years, one "grocer's eczema all his life till lately." *Psoriasis.*—1 case, alternating with asthma. *Varix.*—1 case, many years. *Ulcer of Leg.*—4 cases; one "20 years, now healed," one "for 30 years," one "from 60 to 80, now healed."

ACCIDENTS.—175 returns.   None, 128.

Concussion of Brain.—3 cases; one at 62 and one at 70; the third "four times, was bled each time." *Spinal Concussion.*— 1 case at 34. *Severe Railway Accident.*—one case at 56.— *Knocked Down.*—1 case at 76. *Severe Fall.*—1 case, three weeks ago, scalp wound healed rapidly. *Run Over.*—1 case, by a cab at 80. *Severe Bruising.*—1 case at 64. *Kick on Head.*—1 case when young, large depression of right frontal bone. *Fracture of Skull.*—1 case at 49. *Injury to Chest.*— 1 case at 16, with repeated hæmoptysis and venesection. *Injured Abdomen.*—15 years ago, diarrhœa since.

Dislocation: Shoulder.—6 cases; two at 65 and 79; three 1, 8, and 40 years ago. *Ankle.*—2 cases; one at 50, one 50 years ago. *Hip.*—1 case, 20 years ago. *Injured Hip.*—1 case at 71, lame since.

Fracture: Patella.—2 cases; one 8 months ago, one "muscular at 78, with bony union." *Arm and Leg.*—1 case at 45. *Arm.*—1 case at 83. *Leg and Thigh.*—1 case at 86.: *Right Humerus.*—1 case at 85. *Ribs.*—5 cases; three at 64, 70 and 70, one a year ago with recovery in 3 weeks, one "3 ribs at 58." *Sternum.*—1 case at 30. *Shoulder.*—1 case, "compound, after 70." *Leg.*—2 cases; one at 45. *Thigh.*—6 cases; one 5 years ago, one "in 1880, close to knee," one "left, at 66," one "at 83, in bed nine weeks with perfect union," two of neck of thighbone, one of them in January, 1883, the other "at 79, recovered after being in bed nine weeks."

Amputation: Arm.—1 case at 47. *Leg.*—2 cases; one for "diseased ankle at 25," one from "accident at 46."

LONGEVITY IN FAMILY.—Taking as a standard of a long-lived family one in which of the near relations (grandparents, parents, brothers, sisters, and subject of inquiry) 4 attained the age of 70, or 3 the age of 80, we have at least 182 cases; two of them were on mother's side only; one was returned as short-lived family.

BLOOD-RELATIONSHIP BETWEEN PARENTS OR GRANDPARENTS. —163 returns. None, 157. In two cases "grandparents were cousins," in one "maternal grandparents were first cousins," in one "paternal grandparents were cousins," in one "parents were cousins," in one "parents were first cousins."

AGE OF FATHER AT BIRTH OF SUBJECT OF INQUIRY.—96 returns. *Average*, about 36 years of age.

AGE OF MOTHER AT BIRTH OF SUBJECT OF INQUIRY.—96 returns. *Average*, about 31 years of age.

Only those cases are included in which both age of father and mother are given.

DISEASES IN FAMILY.

Cancer (malignant growths).—44 families.

Consumption.—65 families.

Scrofula.—1 family.

Gout.—30 families.

Apoplexy and Paralysis after 40.—42 families.

Rheumatism.—59 families.

Epilepsy.—5 families.

Insanity.—13 families.

None.—40 families.

NO. III.

ANALYSIS OF RETURNS RELATING TO PRESENT CONDITION,
HABITS, CIRCUMSTANCES, ETC.

Of MALES, from 90 to 100.

92 Returns.

Single, Married, Widowed.—76 returns; S. 4, M. 18, W. 54.

Affluent, Comfortable, Poor.—77 returns; A. 6, C. 42, P. 29.

Fat, Spare, Average.—78 returns; F. 8, Sp. 35, A. 35.

Full-Blooded, Pale, Average.—73 returns; F. 12, P. 16, A. 45.

Strong, Feeble, Average.—76 returns; S. 31, F. 31, A. 14.

Height.—70 returns; average, 5 feet 6⅔ inches; one, now 5 feet 6 inches, was 5 feet 9 inches; another, now 5 feet 5 inches, was 5 feet 7½ inches.

Weight.—39 returns; average, 10 stone 9 pounds.

Figure.—70 returns; erect, 40; bent, 30.

Voice.—76 returns; loud, 10; clear, 10; loud and clear, 33; clear and full, 7; full, 3; loud and full, 2; weak, 5; clear and weak, 6.

Sight.—61 returns; good, 50; *Cataract* (both eyes), 4, in one case at 88 years. *Cataract* (one eye), 1. Failure, apparently independent of presbyopia, 6; in one case "blind for 20 years."

Glasses.—49 returns; none, 10; 39 wore them; of those in which period was given, many years, 3; 2 to 3 years, 1; 8 to 10 years, 5; 12 to 15 years, 4; 16 to 20 years, 6; 26 to 30 years, 5; 40 years, 3; 50 years, 2. In two cases "can read for five minutes without spectacles, and then 'goes all of a piece.'"

Hearing.—77 returns; good, 38; indifferent, 20; bad, 19.

Joints.—77 returns; natural, 64; deformed, 7; stiff, 4; stiff and flexed, 1; stiff and deformed, 1.

Digestion.—74 returns; good, 57; moderate, 14; bad, 3.

Appetite.—74 returns; good, 52; moderate, 17; bad, 5.

Eater.—71 returns; large, 12; moderate, 46; small, 13.

Number of Meals.—55 returns; average rather over 3 each daily.

Alcohol.—73 returns; none, 21; little, 26; moderate, 26; 1 "takes occasionally a little too much."

Animal Food.—69 returns; none, 1; little, 41; moderate, 26; much, 1.

Bowels.—74 returns; daily, 49; three times daily, 1; alternately, 8; every third day, 1; irregular, 13; costive, 2.

Aperients.—72 returns; never, 24; occasionally, 1; frequently, 10; rarely, 37.

Disposition.—76 returns; lethargic, 1; energetic, 28; placid, 28; irritable, 12; placid and energetic, 3; irritable and energetic, 4.

Intellect.—72 returns; high, 12; average, 51; low, 9.

Memory, Past Events.—70 returns; good, 58; moderate, 5; bad, 7.

Memory, Recent Events.—60 returns; good, 34; moderate, 14; bad, 12.

Habits.—75 returns; active, 46; sedentary, 21; bedridden, 8, one for 1 year, one for 2 years.

Out-of-Door Exercise.—68 returns; none, 17, of which 8 were bedridden, 1 not out for years, 1 not for 9 years; little, 7; moderate, 2, one travels by train alone; much, 3, one of these attended Norwich market as a cattle dealer a few days before death, another works in garden 3 hours daily; short walks, 23; walk and drive, 2; walks 1 hour, 1; walks 2 to 3 hours, 1; walk one mile, 3, one of these could do so "easily at 94;" walk 2 miles, 2; walk 3 miles, 3; rides on horseback, 1; "work as labourers," 2; "works on farm," 1; one "at work in hayfield 3 days before death."

Sleep.—70 returns; good, 47; moderate 16; bad, 7.

Sleep, Number of Hours.—39 returns; average, $8\frac{3}{4}$ hours.

Hour of Going to Bed.—54 returns; average, 8.30 P.M.

Hour of Rising.—56 returns; average, 8 A.M.

Chest Girth in Inspiration.—30 returns; average, $35\frac{1}{3}$ inches.

Chest Girth in Expiration.—30 returns; average, 35 inches. Only those cases are included in which chest girth in both inspiration and expiration are given.

Elasticity of Rib Cartilages.—41 returns; distinct, 16; indistinct, 25.

Pulse.—57 returns; average, little over 75 per minute. *Regular, Irregular.*—51 returns; R. 38, I. 13. *Large, Small.* —49 returns; L. 20, S. 29. *Compressible, Incompressible.*—51 returns, C. 42, I. 9.

Arteries.—55 returns; even, 38; visible, 1; visible and even, 2; tortuous, 1; tortuous and even, 2; tortuous and

H. C.   12

visible, 5; knotty, 3; visible and knotty, 2; tortuous and knotty, 1. So they were *visible* in 10 cases, *even* in 42 cases, *tortuous* in 9 cases, *knotty* in 6 cases.

Respiration Number.—48 returns; average, about 23 per minute. *Regular, Irregular.*—48 returns; R. 43, I. 5.

Arcus Senilis.—55 returns; much, 13; little, 22; absent, 20.

Teeth.—69 returns; average, 4 to 5; but 27 had none, and two had "several," one had a "third set of bicuspids at 89 years of age[1];" in 62 cases the teeth are specified. *Upper Incisors*, 44; *canines*, 23; *molars*, 57. *Lower incisors*, 60; *canines*, 40; *molars*, 58.

Artificial Teeth.—71 returns; 66 did not use them, and of these 26 had no teeth, and several others very few; 5 used them; one for 3 years, one for 10 years, one for 20 years.

Evidences of Failure.—58 returns; none, 18; heart, 1; heart and brain, 1; heart and urinary organs, 2; lungs, 9; lungs and urinary organs, 2; lungs, brain, and urinary organs, 1; brain, 4; brain and urinary organs, 1; urinary organs, 19; so the *heart* was affected in 4 cases, the *lungs* in 12 cases, the *brain* in 7 cases, the *urinary organs* in 25 cases. Heart sounds returned as "normal" in 7 cases.

Micturition.—58 returns; natural, 32; slow, 8; frequent, 5; incontinence, 4, one partial for 18 years; difficult, 3, in one case catheter used occasionally, in one from contraction of urethra after amputation of penis. Slow and difficult, 4; slow and frequent, 1; slow, difficult, frequent, and painful, 1; in this case "micturition has been frequent for several years, sometimes a quarter of an hour before he can make water."

---

[1] Probably, as in other instances in which a similar statement has been made, some stumps of old teeth, which had become covered up by the gums, reappeared.

Present Maladies.—63 returns; none, 25.

Debility.—10 cases. *Weak Heart.*—1. *Mitral Bruit.*—1. *Senile Decay.*—1; died. *Cardiac Dropsy.*—1.

Bronchitis.—8 cases; three slight, one for 8 years, one fatal. *Cough.*—2 cases, one chronic. *Emphysema.*—1. *Congestion of Lungs.*—1 case for 2 weeks.

Indigestion.—1. *Ulcer.*—1 from injury. "Gouty erysipelas and eczema."—1 case. *Hernia.*—1 case. *Dementia.*—2 cases; one for a few years, one since 1847 in St Luke's.

Hemiplegia.—1 case. *Brain impaired.*—recently in 1, from anxiety.

Senile Gangrene.—2 cases; 1 of foot, 1 of toe; both died. *Rheumatism.*—4 cases; 1 often, 1 of hip.

Enlarged Prostate.—1 case. *Albuminuria.*—One case for 6 months. *Atony of Bladder.*—One case for 14 years, with occasional retention. *Uræmia* and death, 1 case, difficult micturition from contraction of urethral orifice after amputation of penis for epithelioma 24 years previously.

Temperature.—3 returns; one of 95·0°, two of 96·0°; one of these "under the tongue."

12—2

ANALYSIS RELATING TO PAST HISTORY, INCLUDING FAMILY HISTORY.

Of MALES, from 90 TO 100.

92 Returns.

Age when Married.—62 returns; average, 30 to 31 years of age.

Duration of Married Life.—54 returns; average, little over 47 years.

Number of Children.—68 returns; average, little over 7 each.

Affluent, Comfortable, Poor.—72 returns; A. 6, C. 42, P. 24.

First or —— Child of Parents.—64 returns; 18 are marked "first child," and of these one at least was "only child." In 19 cases the number in the family was also returned; of these, the average position was about third, and the average number of the family was 7 to 8 children. One was a twin, the second born of the two, the other being a girl.

Delicate, Robust, Average.—69 returns; D. 2, R. 47, A. 20.

Health: Good, Moderate.—70 returns; G. 79, M. 9.

Digestion.—74 returns; good, 72; indifferent, 2.

Bowels.—68 returns; good (daily), 58; irregular, 3; costive, 6; loose, 1.

Baldness.—38 returns; early, 12; late, 26.

Greyness.—50 returns; early 13; late, 37.

Disposition.—68 returns; placid, 18; irritable, 5; lethargic, 1; energetic, 32; irritable and energetic, 6; placid and ener- getic, 6.

Intellect.—59 returns; high, 13; average, 44; low, 2.

Habits.—72 returns; active, 70; sedentary, 2.

Out-of-Door Exercise.—68 returns; little, 5; moderate, 6. One "worked hard, often late at night;" one was a "good walker." Much, 57; of these, six were great walkers, one "walking four to five miles daily till 87;" one "ten to twenty miles daily, at 80 could run two miles without stopping;" one "on horseback till 85;" one a "sportsman," one had "laborious occupation;" one "worked hard, often late at night;" one "had a good deal of night-work;" one "often had night-work as a coastguard;" one "a cattle-dealer, often twelve hours without food."

Hours in Bed.—44 returns; average, $8\frac{1}{4}$ hours.

Hour of Rising.—53 returns; average, 6 A.M.

Sleeper.—67 returns; good, 61; average, 4; bad, 2.

Appetite.—67 returns; good, 65; indifferent, 2.

Eater.—66 returns; large, 13; average, 48; small, 5.

Alcohol.—67 returns; none, 1; little, 27; moderate, 32; one of these "took much when he had the chance;" much, 7; of these two were "free eaters and drinkers," one "took two glasses of beer and four glasses of wine daily," one "took three glasses of whisky a day," one was "often drunk and in gaol," one was "drunk about once a week," one "boasted that he smoked and drank more than any man in the town, and was most irregular in every way."

Animal Food.—58 returns; none, 1; little, 14; one of them "once a week;" moderate, 41; much, 2.

ILLNESSES UNDERGONE.—69 returns; none, 32.

"*Fever*"[1] (typhoid?).—6 cases; at 18, 21, 33 severe, 40, 65, and 76. *Typhoid Fever.*—4 cases; one young, three at 45, 50, and 67. *Yellow Fever.*—1 in West Indies. *Typhus Fever.*—4 cases; one at 15, one at 45, one when young in the Peninsular war, one at 65. *Ague.*—1. *Erysipelas.*—4 cases; one at 60, one severe at 80, one severe, with recovery at 89. *Brain Fever.*—1 underwent much venesection.

Bronchitis.—8 cases; three at 80, 88, and 96, one had two attacks in last four years, one severe at 94 with ultimate recovery, one at 98 severe with recovery. *Pneumonia.*—2 cases; one at 75, one within last 4 years.

Phthisis.—1 had symptoms, and at 15 was at Brompton Hospital. *Abscess.*—1 in back at 45.

Jaundice.—2 cases; one at 60, one when young. *Fistula.* —1 at 48.

Epithelioma of Penis.—1 with amputation at 70.

Rheumatism.—2 cases, one as a boy. *Glaucoma.*—1 case, in left eye.

Strangulated Hernia.—1, with operation at 84. *Gangrene.* —1 of left foot at 77. *Venesection.*—1, several times when young.

Eczema.—2 cases; one acute at 90, with complete recovery.

Dementia.—1 case since 1847, in St Luke's.

One had slight paralysis at 72, one slight apoplexy and hemiplegia at 89, one 3 "strokes" with temporary paralysis, one of these during last 15 years also had occasional loss of consciousness and use of left side, with quick recovery.

Retention.—One 4 years ago. *Atony of Bladder.*—One for 14 years from over-distension, occasionally catheterised; one

---

[1] Those designated "*Fever*" and "*Typhus*" were probably in some cases "*Typhoid.*"

for several years has had frequent micturition, sometimes a quarter of an hour before he can make water.

SLIGHT AILMENTS.—63 returns; none, 38.

Bronchitis.—3 cases; one slight, one chronic for 8 years. *Asthma.*—1 case.

Rheumatism.—5 cases; one slight, one at 80, unable to walk since. *Gout.*—4; one for 20 years.

Diarrhœa.—1 lately. *Piles.*—1 for 70 years. *Bilious.*—1. *Ague.*—1. *Gravel.*—1. *Renal Hœmorrhage.*—one case, copious 4 times in last 20 years.

Dizziness.—2 cases; one occasionally for 10 years.

Hernia.—3 cases; one "all life," two for 20 and 50 years.

Ulcer of Leg.—1 case, healed at 98. *Eruption on Legs.* —1. *Eczema.*—1. *Ailing in Youth.*—1.

ACCIDENTS.—49 returns; none, 35.

Concussion.—1 at 84 from fall of 10 feet. *Dislocated Thumb.*—1 from fall from scaffold at 81, recovered. *Sprained Ankle.*—1 at 98, quick recovery. *Scalp Wound.*—2 cases; one severe lately with quick recovery, one from fall at 89, healed quickly.

Fracture: Ribs.—3 cases; one at 84 with speedy recovery, one at 93 healed well. *Clavicle.*—Spontaneous at 90 in raising himself from chair, united. *Thigh.*—1 at 82. *Humerus.*— 1 at 92, perfect union. *Neck of Thighbone.*—2 cases; one 87 not united, one at 20 at Quatre Bras. *Leg.*—4 cases; one at 85, one compound, one both bones at 80 with recovery, one at 80 in middle, "leg slipped off fender as he sat, he did not fall, not united, quite flexible, in bed 7 weeks."

Family Longevity.—Taking as a standard of a long-lived family, one in which of the near relations (grandparents, parents, brothers, sisters, and subject of inquiry) 4 attained the age of

70, or 3 the age of 80, we have at least 40 cases; one was returned as of "short-lived family."

Blood Relationship between Parents or Grandparents.—29 returns; none, 29.

Age of Father at Birth of Subject of Inquiry.—11 returns; average, 35 years of age.

Age of Mother at Birth of Subject of Inquiry.—11 returns; average, nearly 32 years of age. Only those cases are included in which the ages of both father and mother are returned.

Diseases in Family.—*Cancer* (malignant growths).—8 families. *Consumption.*—13 families. *Scrofula.*—0 families. *Gout.*—8 families. *Apoplexy and Paralyses after* 40. — 9 families. *Rheumatism.* — 10 families. *Epilepsy.*—0 families. *Insanity.*—5 families. *None.* —5 families.

In one case almost every member of family except the subject terribly addicted to drink; in another case his son, daughter, and 4 nephews and nieces were deaf mutes.

ANALYSIS OF RETURNS RELATING TO PRESENT CONDITION,
HABITS, CIRCUMSTANCES, ETC.

Of WOMEN from 80 to 90.

282 Returns.

Single, Married, Widowed.—280 returns; S. 32, M. 26, W.
222.

Affluent, Comfortable, Poor.—280 returns; A. 23, C. 112,
P. 145.

Fat, Spare, Average.—277 returns; F. 36, S. 119, A. 122.

Full-blooded, Pale, Average.—275 returns; F. 18, P. 104,
A. 153.

Strong, Feeble, Average.—274 returns; S. 58, F. 110, A.
106.

Height.—218 returns; average, a little over 5 feet 2 inches.

Weight.—86 returns; average, about 8 stone 10½ pounds.

Figure.—242 returns; erect, 146 ; bent, 96.

Voice.—268 returns; clear, 103 ; loud, 40; weak, 32; full,
11 ; clear and weak, 9; clear and full, 23 ; loud and clear, 49;
loud and full, 1.

Sight.—220 returns; good, 184 ; cataracts, 15 ; failure apparently independent of presbyopia, 21.

Glasses.—227 returns; none, 32 ; 195 wore them.   In
some the number of years during which they were worn was

given; many years, 19; 2 to 3 years, 2; 4 to 5 years, 6; 6 to 7 years, 4; 8 to 10 years, 14; 12 to 15 years, 10; 16 to 20 years, 31; 21 to 25 years, 10; 26 to 30 years, 34; 31 to 35 years, 6; 36 to 40 years, 28; 41 to 45 years, 3; 46 to 50 years, 10; 54 years, 1; 58 years, 1; 60 years, 1; 65 years, 1.

Hearing.—279 returns; good, 175; indifferent, 77; bad, 27.

Joints.—278 returns; natural, 243; stiff, 12; deformed, 13; stiff and deformed, 10.

Digestion.—280 returns; good, 169; moderate, 94; bad, 17.

Appetite.—278 returns; good, 144; moderate, 115; bad, 19.

Eater.—275 returns; large, 22; small, 105; moderate, 148.

Number of Meals.—225 returns; average, 3 to 4 daily.

Alcohol.—270 returns; none, 105; little, 117; moderate, 44; much, 4.

Animal Food.—249 returns; none, 10; little, 164; moderate, 72; much, 3.

Bowels.—266 returns; daily, 183; irregular, 51; alternately, 30; costive, 1; once a week, 1.

Aperients.—265 returns; never, 58; rarely, 150; frequently, 52; daily, 3; occasionally, 2.

Disposition.—267 returns; placid, 119; irritable, 28; lethargic, 4; energetic, 93; placid and energetic, 14; irritable and energetic, 9.

Intellect.—266 returns; high, 33; low, 36; average, 197.

Memory, Past Events.—258 returns; good, 186; moderate, 41; bad, 31. *Recent Events.*—221 returns; good, 120; moderate, 58; bad, 43.

Habits.—275 returns; active, 128; sedentary, 100; bedridden, 47; of these five for 2, 3, 4, 4, 15 years respectively, and two for 3 weeks and 3 months respectively.

Out-of-Door Exercise.—252 returns; none, 88 (of these 47 were bedridden); little, 102; moderate, 34; much, 14; short walks, 18 (of these one walks 2 miles). Besides these, three walk 3, 4 and 6 miles respectively.

Sleep.—267 returns; good, 146; moderate, 89; bad, 32.

Number of Hours.—147 returns; average, a little over 7 hours.

Hours of Going to Bed.—204 returns; average, a little past 9 o'clock P.M.

Hour of Rising.—202 returns; average, 7.45 A.M.

Chest Girth in Inspiration.—73 returns; average, about $31\frac{1}{4}$ inches. *Expiration.*—73 returns; average, about $30\frac{1}{2}$ inches. Only those are included where both inspiration and expiration are given.

Elasticity of Rib Cartilages.—139 returns; distinct, 65; indistinct, 74.

Pulse.—228 returns; average, nearly 79 per minute; high, owing to chest affections in many cases. *Regular, Irregular.*—201 returns; R. 164, I. 37. *Large, Small.*—194 returns; L. 60, S. 134. *Compressible, Incompressible.*—221 returns; C. 181, I. 40.

Arteries.—211 returns; even, 138; visible, 13; tortuous and even, 8; visible and even, 11; tortuous, 13; tortuous and visible, 6; knotty, 6; visible and knotty, 2; tortuous and knotty, 12; tortuous, visible, and knotty, 1; tortuous, visible, and even, 1; so that they were *even* in 158 cases, *tortuous* in 41 cases, *visible* in 34 cases, *knotty* in 21 cases.

Respiration.—Number, 204 returns; average, nearly 22 per minute; rather high, owing to chest complaints in many cases. *Regular, Irregular.*—212 returns; R. 198, I. 14.

Arcus Senilis.—224 returns; much, 48; little, 80; absent, 96.

Teeth.—253 returns; average, little over 3 each; but 122 had no teeth; of these, two had not had any for 40 and 55 years respectively. In 241 cases the teeth were specified. *Upper incisors*, 103; *canines*, 75; *molars*, 96. *Lower incisors*, 201; *canines*, 112; *molars*, 121.

Artificial Teeth.—208 returns; none, 176; of these, 89 had not any teeth, and 4 had not had any for 4, 30, 40, and 40 years respectively, and 3 had not had any "for years," and many others had very few teeth; 32 used artificial teeth, in some cases the number of years during which they had been worn was given. Many years, 5; 5 years, 1; 7 years, 1; 10 years, 2; 12 years, 1; 15 years, 1; 20 years, 4; 21 years, 1; 25 years, 3; 30 years, 4; 36 years, 1; 40 years, 1; 55 years (full set), 1.

Evidences of Failure.—228 returns; none, 117; heart, 11; heart and lungs, 6; heart and brain, 5; heart and urinary organs, 5; heart, lungs, and urinary organs, 2; heart, brain, and urinary organs, 2; heart, lungs, brain, and urinary organs, 5; in 14 cases heart-sounds returned as normal; lungs, 21; lungs and brain, 3; lungs and urinary organs, 7; brain, 18; brain and urinary organs, 3; urinary organs, 23; so that the *heart* was affected in 36 cases, the *lungs* in 44 cases, the *brain* in 36 cases, the *urinary organs* in 47 cases; in the case of the urinary organs, the failure was often slight (*vide* Micturition).

Micturition.—207 returns; natural, 166; incontinence, 13; slow, 11; slow and difficult, 3; frequent, 8; painful, 1; difficult 1; hæmaturia, 1; difficult and painful, 1; slow, difficult, and painful, 2.

PRESENT MALADIES.—248 returns; none 91. *Debility.*—34 cases. *Weak Heart.*—5. *Syncope.*—2. *Palpitations.*—3. *Ver-*

tigo.—3. *Angina.*—1, occasionally. *"Aortic Disease."*—1. *Murmur at Base.*—2 cases, one of them systolic.

Dyspepsia.—9. *Diarrhœa.*—5, one slight, one occasionally. *Piles.*—3. *Flatulence.*—2. *Constipation.*—1. *Hernia.* —5, one for 40 years, one strangulated, with death three days after herniotomy, one umbilical.

Bronchitis.—32 cases, 6 of them chronic. *Cough.*—2. *Emphysema.*—2. *Pneumonia.*--1.

Rheumatism, Rheumatic Gout.—26 cases. *Gout.*—6. *Swelled Knee.*—1.

Uterine Hæmorrhage.—1. *Polypus Uteri.*—1. *Prolapsus Uteri.*—4, one for 30 years. *Irritable Bladder.*—2. *Retention of Urine.*—1. *Intermittent Hæmaturia.*—1, for 20 years.

Caries of Rib.—1. *Lame (Hip).*—1. *Diseased Ankle.*—1, for many years. *Fracture of Neck of Femur.*—2.

Cancer of Breast.—5. *Epithelioma of Face.*—1. *Rodent Cancer.*—1. *Carbuncle.*—1, large. *Periostitis.*—1.

Eczema.—3. *Erythema of Leg.*—1. *Sore Eyes.*—3. *Sore Mouth.*—1. *Eczema of Nipple.*—1 (no cancer). *Ulcer of Leg.* —1. *Inflamed Legs.*—1.

Neuralgia (Face).—3. *Sciatica.*—2. *Lumbago.*—1. *Hysteria.*—1. *Paralysis Agitans.*—2. *"Lunatic."*—1. *Dementia.* —13 cases. Besides these, one with epileptic attacks, and occasional delusions and excitement, and one "light-headed for one year." *Epilepsy.*—1, occasionally. *Mania.*—1, chronic; well for 17 years, recurring at 57.

Hemiplegia.—6. *Paraplegia.*—1. *Paralysis of Left Arm.* —1. *Senile Fits.*—1.

Temperature.—6 returns; in two cases "normal;" in three, 98·0°; in one, 98·2°.

ANALYSIS OF RETURNS RELATING TO PAST HISTORY, INCLUDING FAMILY HISTORY.

Of FEMALES, from 80 to 90.

282 Returns.

Age when Married.—220 returns ; average, about 26 years of age.

Duration of Married Life.—199 returns; average, nearly 39½.

Number of Children.—228 returns ; average, 5 to 6 each, but 43 had no children ; one had " prostration at 41, from child-bearing," one " often ailing since a bad labour 46 years ago," one " had severe flooding at 42, with difficulty rallying," one " nursed 8 children for a year each," two " many miscarriages," one " 7 miscarriages out of 10 conceptions," one had " only one child, still-born," one " early profuse catamenia, menopause at 48," one " catamenia commencing at 16, moderate," one " catamenia from 17 to 40, moderate."

Affluent, Comfortable, Poor.—263 returns ; A. 23, C. 138, P. 102.

First or — Child of Parents.—249 returns ; average about 4th child. In 70 cases the number in the family was returned ; in these the average position was 3rd to 4th, and the average number in the family 7 to 8 children ; 58 were " first child," and of these 4 at least were "only child;" three were twins, and two twin brothers of one of the subjects both died over 80 years old; the mother of one not included in above had 22 children, and the maternal grandmother of one included above had 22 children, of whom 20 grew up.

Delicate, Robust, Average.—240 returns; D. 37, R. 100, A. 103.

Health.—232 returns; good, 207; moderate, 25.

Often Ailing, Rarely Ailing.—26 returns; O. 25, R. 1.

Digestion.—248 returns; good, 211; indifferent, 37.

Bowels.—226 returns; regular, 184; irregular, 9; costive, 29; relaxed, 3; twice daily, 1.

Baldness.—80 returns; early, 17; late, 61; none, 2.

Greyness.—210 returns; early, 53; late, 155; none, 2.

Disposition.—242 returns; placid, 74; irritable, 20; lethargic, 2; energetic, 128; irritable and energetic, 13; placid and energetic, 5.

Intellect.—238 returns; high, 43; average, 180; low, 15.

Habits.—234 returns; active, 215; sedentary, 19.

Out-of-Door Exercise.—206 returns; little, 64; moderate, 72, one a moderate walker; much, 59, one hard, working. Besides these, eleven others: one worked hard, one walked daily, one "good walker," one "walked 3 hours," five "took walks," one "could walk 30 to 40 miles when young," one was "never very active."

Hours in Bed.—171 returns; average a little over 8 hours.

Hour of Rising.—196 returns; average a little past 6 A.M.

Sleeper.—232 returns; good, 188; average, 33; bad, 11.

Appetite.—233 returns; good, 209; indifferent, 24.

Eater.—230 returns; large, 29; small, 63; average, 138.

Alcohol.—232 returns; none, 54; very little, 2; little, 109, one of these "none till 35;" moderate, 60, one of these "none till 40;" much, 7, one of these was a "notorious drinker, locked up 200 times for being drunk, father died aged 90, and brother died aged 70, both heavy drinkers."

ILLNESSES UNDERGONE.—231 returns; none, 111.

"*Fever.*" [1]—19 cases; three "young," two severe at 20 and 60, eight at 28, 30, 50, 60, 40, 60, 63, and 70 respectively. *Measles.*—1 case. *Tonsillitis.*—1 case. *Typhus Fever.*—10 cases; 1 "young," five at 15, 20, 28, 30, and 46 respectively. *Scarlet Fever.*—5 cases; two severe at 40 and 42; one at 72. *Typhoid Fever.*—6 cases; one at 42 severe, five at 12, 19, 30, 47, and 70 respectively. *Influenza.*—1 case at 68. *Croup.*—1 case at 16, was bled excessively. *Whooping-cough.*—1 case. *Erysipelas.*—5 cases; "frequently" one and severe at 57, three of face at 20, 57, and 62 respectively. *Diphtheria.*—1 case at 68. *Rheumatic Fever.*—14 cases; one twice, one prolonged at 74, one at 26, deaf since; five at 21, 24, 26, 30, and 72 respectively. *Rheumatism.*—3 cases. *Gout.*—3 cases; at 31, 73, and 81. *Sunstroke*—1 case at 52. *Cholera.*—1 case at 30. *Dysentery.*—1 case, severe, at 50.

Jaundice.—4 cases; three at 12, 81, and 83; all recovering. *Enteritis.*—4 cases; two at 44 and 80, one severe at 34. *Hæmatemesis.*—1 case at 60. *Diarrhœa.*—2 cases; one at 88 severe, recovered. *Bilious Attacks.*—2 cases; one at 60, with gall-stones; one "severe to point of sinking." *Gall-stones.*—2 cases; one "badly when young." *Gall-stones and Jaundice.*—1 case at 66. *Inflammation of Liver.*—1 case at 73. *Strangulated Hernia.*—2 cases, at 50 and 85, with death in latter. *Intestinal Obstruction*, 1 case at 76.

Pneumonia.—7 cases; one at 82, recovered; one at 72, with pleurisy; one severe at 69, and four at 57, 67, 79, and

---

[1] Some of those designated "*Fever*" and "*Typhus*" were probably "*Typhoid.*"

80.   *Congestion of Lungs.*—1 case at 83.   *Pleurisy.*—6 cases;
five at 20, 40, 50, 60, and 72.   *Bronchitis.*—26 cases; five at
25, 81, 86, "86 for four months," and "after 80" respectively;
four severe at 62, 74, 80, and 88 respectively; two died; one
6 months ago; three "winter bronchitis" (one of them for
5 years); one 15 years ago, one at "80 with complete
recovery," one 3 severe attacks at 76, 77, 78; one with
pneumonia at 86 recovering; one had "two attacks in last 2
years."

   Uterine Fibroid.—1 case.   *Nephritis.*—1 case at 77.   *Phle-
bitis.*—case at 75 recovering.   *Gangrene.*—1 case at 75 recovering.   *Herpes.*—1 case at 77 never completely recovering.
Glaucoma, with removal of eye.—1 case.   *Feeble Heart and
Anasarca.*—1 case for several years.   *Poisoned Hand.*—1 case,
12 years ago; laid up several months.   *"Inflammation."*—1
case at 30.   *Abscess.*—1 case in thigh at 57.   *Eczema.*—1 case
for 2 years at 78; one "three years at 50."

   Insanity.—1 case.   *Paralysis Agitans.*—1 case at 66.   *Paralysis.*—2 cases at 79 recovering, and 82.   *Hemiplegia.*—8 cases;
one 2 years ago, one 3 years ago for a week, two at 81 and 82,
both recovering; two at 77 and 78, with "partial recovery;"
and two at 72 and 81.

   Cancer of Breast.—3 cases; two doubtful and removed, one
of them at 50, the third, "from injury 16 years before death,
did not trouble her until ulcer of leg healed one year before
her death."

   SLIGHT AILMENTS.—218 returns.   None, 119.

   Dyspepsia.—21 cases; one for 5 years, 1 "all her life."
Bilious Attacks.—3 cases.   *Piles.*—4 cases.   *"Spasms."*—1 case.
Congestion of Liver.—2 cases.   *Costive.*—1 case, since typhoid
fever at 47.   *Diarrhœa.*—2 cases; one occasionally.

   H. C.   13

Headaches.—7 cases; one "all her life," one "terrible from 20 to 50 years of age." *Pruritus.*—1 case for 40 years. *Neuralgia.*—1 case.

Palpitations.—4 cases; 1 "all her life," 1 for many years. *Menorrhagia.*—1 case. *Amenorrhœa.*—1 case. *Hysteria.*—1 case. *Prolapsus Uteri.*—2 cases. *Hernia.*—5 cases; three for many, 20, and 40 years; one "femoral" for 15 years; one large umbilical.

Gout.—5 cases; one frequently, one "for 15 years."

Rheumatism.—16 cases; one for 20 years, one since 76 years of age.

Bronchitis.—14 cases; one "slight, occasionally," one "not for 10 years," one "for 10 years." *Coughs.*—2 cases; one for many years. *Catarrhs.*—1 case.

Eczema.—1 case. *Sore Leg.*—1 case. *Œdema of Legs.*—1 case, recently. *Ulcer of Leg.*—4 cases; one for 8 years.

Hæmaturia.—2 cases; one in "3 successive springs," one "intermittent for 20 years." *Lame.*—1 case "from birth."

Melancholy.—1 case. *Debility.*—1 case. *Delicate.*—2 cases; one "throughout life," one "in early life." *Lateral Curvature.*—1 case. One took $\frac{2}{3}$th grain of morphine daily for many years.

ACCIDENTS.—188 returns. None, 150.

Burn.—1 case, "when a child." *Concussion of Brain.*—1 case at 36. *Head injury.*—1 case at 79. *Jarred* by railway accident.—1 case, 30 years ago. *Injury to Back.*—2 cases; one at 35; one from fall, bedridden since. *Fall Downstairs.*—3 cases; one at 88, one 2 years ago; her pulse, previously 60, has been 120 per minute since.

Amputation: Leg.—1 case at 50, for accident. *Breast.*—2 cases; for doubtful cancer, one at 50; one recovered in 14

days (*Lancet*, June, 1885). "*Operation for Tumour of Womb.*"
—1 case at 53. *Herniotomy.*—1 case; death, 3 days later.
Dislocation of Shoulder.—3 cases, two at 70 and 79.
Fracture: Neck of Femur.—6 cases; one 4 years ago, one
"3 years ago, bedridden since;" four at 70, 81, 81, and "77
with recovery[1]." *Thigh.*—3 cases; two at 40 and 74, one 9
months ago (*Lancet*, April, 1884). *Arm.*—5 cases, at 6, 60,
78, 80, "70, with quick recovery." *Forearm.*—2 cases; at 84,
and "82, with firm union in 25 days." *Wrist.*—1 case; in one
wrist at 60 and in the other at 78. *Ribs.*—5 cases; three at
25, 60 and 81. *Patella.*—1 case at 25. *Hip.*—1 case at 57,
on crutches since. *Both Legs.*—1 case at 78. *Compound Fracture of Leg.*—1 case 10 years ago, no lameness.

Longevity in Family.—Taking as a standard of a long-lived
family one in which of the near relations (grandparents, parents,
brothers, sisters, and subject of inquiry), 4 attained the age of
70, or 3 the age of 80, we have at least 135 cases. Five
families were returned as "short-lived."

Relationship between Parents or Grandparents.—134 returns. None, 139. Parents, first cousins, 1. Parents, second
cousins, 1.

Age of Father at Birth of Subject of Inquiry.—70 returns;
average, rather over 33½ years of age.

Age of Mother at Birth of Subject of Inquiry.—70 returns;
average, about 29½ years. Only those cases are included in
which the ages of both the father and mother are returned.

Diseases in Family.—*Cancer* (malignant growths).—30

[1] In this, and other cases, where recovery is mentioned, it is stated in
the return to have taken place; but it is not necessarily to be inferred
that recovery did not take place in the instances in which mention of it
is omitted.

13—2

families.   *Consumption.*—75 families.   *Scrofula.*—1 family.
Gout.—24 families.   *Apoplexy and Paralysis after* 40.—45
families.   *Rheumatism.*—53 families.   *Epilepsy.*—3 families.
Insanity.—28 families.   *None.*—21 families[1].

[1] This scarcely enables us to form an estimate respecting the absence
of disease in the families, forasmuch as no return will have been made
in many cases in which disease did not form part of the family-history.

ANALYSIS OF RETURNS RELATING TO PRESENT CONDITION, HABITS, CIRCUMSTANCES, ETC.

Of WOMEN, from 90 to 100.

110 Returns.

Single, Married, Widowed.—108 returns; S. 15, M. 10, W. 83.

Affluent, Comfortable, Poor.—110 returns; A. 12, C. 46, P. 52.

Fat, Spare, Average.—109 returns; F. 10, S. 62, A. 37.

Full-blooded, Pale, Average.—104 returns; F. 7, P. 56, A. 41.

Strong, Feeble, Average.—106 returns; S. 28, F. 45, A. 33.

Height.—92 returns; average, 5 feet $2\frac{1}{4}$ inches.

Weight.—28 returns; average, 8 stone $7\frac{1}{2}$ pounds nearly.

Figure.—93 returns; erect, 54; bent, 39.

Voice.—105 returns; clear, 25; full, 5; loud and clear, 33; weak, 11; clear and full, 14; loud, 11; clear and weak, 6.

Sight.—93 returns; good, 58; cataracts, 12; one at 85, and two for 1 and 4 years respectively. Failure, apparently independent of presbyopia, 23; one blind for 2 years.

Glasses.—77 returns; none, 16; 61 wore them. In many cases the number of years during which they were worn was given. Few years, 1; many years, 9; 4 to 5 years, 2; 8 to

10 years, 2; 12 to 15 years, 1; 16 to 20 years, 6; 21 to 25 years, 2; 26 to 30 years, 6; 31 to 35 years, 3; 36 to 40 years, 10; 41 to 45 years, 3; 46 to 50 years, 6; 60 years, 2; 57 years, 1; 63 years, 1; 75 years, 1; 83 years, 1. Of those who use no glasses, two can thread a needle without; one used them from 40 to 80, but reads well without them now; one used them from 40 to 60, but reads well without them now.

Hearing.—110 returns; good, 48; indifferent, 34; bad, 28.

Joints.—107 returns; natural, 90; deformed, 7; stiff, 5; stiff and deformed, 4; slight Dupuytren's contraction, 1.

Digestion.—107 returns; good, 84; moderate, 21; bad, 2; one can "live on anything, and eat anything."

Appetite.—108 returns; good, 71; moderate, 34; bad, 3.

Eater.—101 returns; large, 10; moderate, 62; small, 29.

Number of Meals.—77 returns; average, 3 to 4 daily.

Alcohol.—105 returns; none, 32; moderate, 24; little, 48; much, 1.

Animal Food.—98 returns; none, 4; moderate, 38; little, 56.

Bowels.—103 returns; once a week, 1; twice daily, 1; alternately, 8; irregular, 22; daily, 71.

Aperients.—97 returns; daily, 2; frequently, 20, in one case the "bowels never acted without;" rarely, 48; never, 27.

Disposition.—105 returns; placid, 37; irritable, 13; lethargic, 2; energetic, 32; irritable and energetic, 14; placid and energetic, 7.

Intellect.—102 returns; high, 18; average, 71; low, 13.

Memory, Past Events.—105 returns; good, 80; moderate, 11; bad, 14.

Memory, Recent Events.—93 returns; good, 55; moderate, 17; bad, 21.

Habits.—108 returns; active, 48; sedentary, 33; bedridden, 27, 2 for a year, 1 for 6 months.

Out-of-door Exercise.—104 returns; none, 50, of whom 27 were bedridden; little, 25; moderate, 2; short walks, 21; one of these "walked 4 miles last week;" walk much, 4; of these, one "able to walk some miles," one "walked 3 miles within a month of her death, and walked a third of a mile to morning service and back on the day before death; died from a cold." Drives out, 1.

Sleep.—103 returns; good, 69; moderate, 24; bad, 10, one of these kept awake by rheumatic pains.

Sleep, Number of Hours.—59 returns; average, about $7\frac{3}{4}$ hours.

Hour of Going to Bed.—71 returns; average, little past 8.30 P.M.

Hour of Rising.—70 returns; average, about 8.45 A.M.

Chest-girth, in Inspiration.—27 returns; average $31\frac{1}{5}$ (about). *Expiration.*—27 returns; average $30\frac{1}{4}$ (about). Only those cases are included in which chest-girth in both inspiration and expiration are returned.

Elasticity of Rib-cartilages.—53 returns; distinct, 28; indistinct, 25.

Pulse Number.—78 returns; average, nearly 80 per minute; high from chest affections in many cases. *Regular, Irregular.* —70 returns; R. 60, I. 10. *Large, Small.*—72 returns; L. 20, S. 52. *Compressible, Incompressible.*—75 returns; C. 63, I. 12.

Arteries.—71 returns; even, 54; tortuous, 1; visible, 1; visible and even, 6; tortuous and visible, 4; tortuous and even, 2; knotty, 1; tortuous and knotty, 1; visible and knotty, 1. So they were *even* in 62 cases, *tortuous* in 8 cases, *visible* in 12 cases, *knotty* in 3 cases.

Respiration Number.—62 returns; average, 21 to 22 per minute; higher from chest affections in many cases. *Regular, Irregular.*—67 returns; R. 65, I. 2.

Arcus Senilis.—77 returns; much, 23; little, 25; absent, 29.

Teeth.—95 returns; average, a little over 2 each, but 58 had no teeth, one "none for 20 years;" one "lost teeth when young, but can eat a beefsteak as well as anyone." In 92 cases the teeth are specified. *Upper incisors*, 26; *canines*, 23; *molars*, 25. *Lower incisors*, 49; *canines*, 26; *molars*, 41.

Artificial Teeth.—96 returns; none, 85; 11 used artificial teeth, and another did so formerly. Of these for many years, 4; "from early life," 1; 10 years, 1; 30 years, 1; 45 years, 1; 50 years, 2.

Evidences of Failure.—83 returns; none, 43; heart, 4; heart and lungs, 1; heart and brain, 1; heart and urinary organs, 2; heart, lungs, and urinary organs, 1; lungs, 3; lungs and urinary organs, 2; brain, 15; urinary organs, 11; so that the *heart* was affected in 9 cases, the *lungs* in 7 cases, the *brain* in 16 cases, the *urinary organs* in 16 cases.

Micturition.—79 returns; natural, 63; slow, 6; frequent, 3; difficult, 2; incontinence, 1; slow and difficult, 1; slow, difficult, and painful, 1; difficult and painful, 1; difficult and frequent, 1.

Heart Sounds returned as "normal" in 13 cases.

PRESENT MALADIES.—86 returns; none, 39.

Bronchitis.—6 cases; 3 slight. *Chronic Cough.*—1. *Weak Heart.*—1. *Syncope.*—1, slight. *Anasarca.*—1, few months. *Œdema.*—3 cases, of legs, ankles, and feet respectively. *Valvular Disease.*—1, long-standing disease; carried up and down stairs for years; breath short. *Murmurs.*—4 cases, 2 "systolic," 1 "basic," 1 "basic systolic."

Debility.—13.   *General Decay and Death.*—2 cases.
Rheumatism.—5.

Abdominal Tumour.—1 case, dying semicomatose soon after.   *Tumour of Right Hypochondrium.*—1 case, for many years.

Diabetes.—1.   *Bilious.*—1.   *Constipation.*—1.

Neuralgia.—2 cases after *herpes*, 1 of arm after herpes a year ago, 1 for 9 months.

Gastralgia.—1.   *Varix of Leg.*—1.   *Ulcer of Leg.*—1, for 2 years.

Tremors.—1.   "*Wanders.*"—1.   "*Excitement and Illusions.*" —1.   "*Childish.*"—2.   *Senile Dementia.*—1.   *Imbecile.*—1. *Slight Paralysis.*—1.   *Senile Paralysis.*—1, for 5 years.   *Epileptic Convulsions.*—1.   *Partial Left Hemiplegia.*—1.   *Apoplexy and Left Hemiplegia,* 1.

ANALYSIS OF RETURNS RELATING TO PAST HISTORY, INCLUDING FAMILY HISTORY.

Of WOMEN, from 90 to 100.
110 Returns.

Age when Married.—72 returns; average, 26 to 27 years of age, and 1 married again at 81 years of age.

Duration of Married Life.—64 returns; average, 42 to 43 years.

Number of Children.—83 returns; average, nearly 6 each, but 14 had no children, 1 of these having been married 3 times; in 1 case all labours (14) instrumental, killing most of children; 1 had 7 children, and of these 2 were twin daughters, both alive at 57 had large families, and 1 had twin boys.

Affluent, Comfortable, Poor.—102 returns; A. 14, C. 50, P. 38.

First or — Child of Parents.—80 returns; average, fourth child; 20 were "first child," and of these at least 1 was an "only child." In 24 cases the number in the family was also given; of these the average position was third to fourth, and the average number in the family 7 to 8.

Delicate, Robust, Average.—95 returns; D. 10, R. 48, A. 37.

Health : Good, Moderate.—95 returns; G. 90, M. 5.

    „   *Often, Rarely Ailing.*—12 returns; O. 10, R. 2.

Digestion.—99 returns; good, 94; indifferent, 5.

Bowels.—88 returns; good, 77; costive, 9; irregular, 2. One "took much aperient medicine till 70;" another "all her life."

Baldness.—27 returns; early, 5, 1 "from eczema;" late, 22. One had much hair on chin.

Greyness.—71 returns; early, 18; late, 53.

Disposition.—97 returns; placid, 26; irritable, 9; energetic, 41; irritable and energetic, 12; placid and energetic, 8; placid and lethargic, 1.

Intellect.—92 returns; high, 23; low, 3; average, 66.

Habits.—140 returns; active, 132; sedentary, 8.

Out-of-door Exercise.—87 returns; little, 19, one a laundress till 92; moderate, 28, one a bad walker; great walkers, 2; much, 38, of these 2 were good walkers and 1 a great walker; 1 "walked barefoot all her life, and does so all the year round;" 1 a "noted tobacco smuggler, many hardships, slept in chair 50 years without undressing."

Hours in Bed.—60 returns; average, about $8\frac{1}{4}$ hours.

Hour of Rising.—74 returns; average, about 6.15 A.M.

Sleeper.—83 returns; good, 75; average, 11; bad, 3.

Appetite.—89 returns; good, 85; indifferent, 4.

Eater.—87 returns; large, 10; average, 56; small 21.

Alcohol.—92 returns; none, 22; very little, 1; little, 43; moderate, 24; rather free, 1; much, 1.

Animal Food.—82 returns; little, 38; moderate, 43; much, 1.

ILLNESS UNDERGONE.—93 returns; none, 42.

"*Fever*[1]."—2 cases; one severe at 30, one "many years ago." *Scarlet Fever.*—1 case, severe at 19. *Typhus Fever.*

---

[1] Some of those designated "*Fever*" and "*Typhus Fever*" were probably "*Typhoid Fever.*"

—2 cases at 27 and 42. *Typhoid Fever.*—1 case at 27. *Croup.* —1 case at 50. *English Cholera.*—1 case at 80. *Smallpox.*—1 case. *Erysipelas.*—3 cases; one severe, one of head.

Chorea.—1 case twice, at 7 and 10. *Rheumatic Fever.*—6 cases; three at 18, 40, 40, two at·50, severe. *Rheumatism.* —3 cases; one at 82 for six months. *Gout.*—2 cases; one occasionally for 16 years.

Diarrhœa.—1 case. *Enteritis.*—2 cases; one at 76, one at 71, with complete recovery. *Hæmatemesis.*—1 at 78 ; no return.

Jaundice.—3 cases; one at 60, one severe at 40. *Congested Liver.*—1 at 88.

Poisoned Hand.—1 at 95. *Sloughing Ulcer of Foot.*—6 months ago, quite healed. *Inflammation in Side.*—1 case, twice. *Pelvic Abscess.*—1 case at 45. *Herpes.*—2 cases : one at 92, one of right side of head and neck at 95.

Bronchitis.—13 cases ; three at 75, 78, and 96 respectively, one "several times," one "lately, severe, with recovery," one "3 times in 20 years," one "severe at 67," one "3 times, at 75, 76, and 89, with recovery from each in 3 months," one "severe at 95, with complete recovery."

Pneumonia.—5 cases; two at 60 and 78, one "double, severe, at 94, with recovery in 6 weeks." *Congestion of Lungs.*—1 at 93. *Spasmodic Asthma.*—1 case, severe from 50 to 70, circumstances then suddenly reduced her from affluence to penury, and the asthma ceased.

Valvular Disease of Heart.—1 case, long standing, short breath, carried up and down stairs for years.

Paralysis.—2 cases ; 1 at 60, complete recovery, one twice, at 85 and 90, with partial recovery. *Apoplexy.*—2 cases ; in one 3 attacks, two at 83, the third at 90 with death.

Paraplegia.—1, two years ago. *Hemiplegia.*—3 cases ; one

right, at 89, recovered use of leg, not of arm ; one had several attacks and recoveries, namely, left hemiplegia and convulsions at 78, with good recovery, paralysis of left hand at 82, severe apoplexy at 89½ ; got about again, but mind weakened and with occasional epileptic attacks. One was "out of her mind" for a few days a short time ago, slept 14 hours, and awoke well.

Slight Ailments.—79 returns; none, 52.

Bronchitis.—3 cases. *Coughs.*—2 cases; one slight, one for 20 years. *Winter Cough.*—1 case.

Indigestion.—1 case, "all her life." *Gastralgia.*—1 case.

Bilious Attacks.—2 cases. *Bilious Headaches.*—2 cases; one when young. *Headaches.*—6 cases; one of "sick headaches," one "severe every month," one "till 60 years old," one "severe till 50 years old."

Diarrhœa.—1 case occasionally.

Gravel.—1 case, slight, lately. *Eczema.*—1 case, slight.

Delicate.—2 cases; one when young. *Neuralgia.*—1 case.

Rheumatism.—2 cases. *Syncope.*—2 cases ; one occasionally.

Conjunctivitis.—2 cases. *Varix of Leg.*—1 case. *Prolapsus Uteri.*—2 cases. *Polypus Uteri.*—1 case.

Irritability of several Mucous Membranes.—1 case, from 40 till death.

Issue for 60 *Years.*—1 case, closed 3 years ago, with gain in weight after.

Frequently in Bed, and Bled because Full-blooded.—1 case.

Accidents.—71 returns ; none, 57.

Falls.—3 ; one "downstairs at 94, sedentary since," and two at 87 and 90 respectively.

Burn.—1 at 92, perfect healing. *Contusion.*—1 severe at 34.

Fracture: Ribs.—1 at 84. *Arm.*—1, 6 years ago, rapid recovery. *Thigh.*—1 at 90. *Colles's.*—1 at 89, rapid union. *Neck of Femur.*—4 cases; one at 93, one died in 3 months, one "10 years ago," one "at 80, not united." *Injury to Hip.*—2 cases, one at 88 with lameness since, one 6 months before death.

Blood-Relationship between Parents or Grandparents.—41 returns; none, 38. Parents, distant relations, 1; cousins, 1; first cousins, 1.

Age of Father at Birth of Subject of Inquiry.—19 returns; average, $32\frac{1}{2}$ years old.

Age of Mother at Birth of Subject of Inquiry.—19 returns; average, nearly 29 years old. Only those cases are included in which the ages of both father and mother are returned.

Diseases in Family. — *Cancer* (malignant growths).— 15 families. *Consumption.*—16 families. *Scrofula.* — 1 family. *Gout.*—9 families. *Apoplexy and Paralysis after* 40.—16 families. *Rheumatism.*—18 families. *Epilepsy.*—2 families. *Insanity.*—8 families. *None.*—11 families.

Longevity in Family.—Taking as a standard of a long-lived family one in which, of the near relations (grandparents, parents, brothers, sisters, and subject of inquiry), 4 attained the age of 70, or 3 the age of 80, we have at least 49 cases.

APPENDIX.

THE accompanying photographs of Benjamin Atkins and Elizabeth his wife, each aged 101, are from a negative taken by the Rev. J. R. Smith, and kindly lent by him. In March, 1889, Mr Amyot of Diss was so good as to send me photographs and some particulars of this old couple. The man died on May 9th; and on August 2nd Dr Barnes of Eye, in Suffolk, kindly drove Mr Amyot and myself a distance of seven miles over to Brockdish to see the survivor. Both she and her husband had taken to bed at the beginning of the winter, rather for the warmth than from inability to get up, and she was still there; a pale, thin, healthy woman with good features and healthy complexion, brisk in movement, quick of hearing, with good sight, very good appetite and digestion, daily action of bowels, pulse 80, arteries firm, breathing quick (40), perhaps increased in rate by the excitement from our visit; heart's sounds natural, teeth all gone; a good covering of grey hair on the head; entirely without ailment except that she is troubled with frequency of micturition, often getting out of bed for the purpose and, on this account, getting very little sleep. Mentally she is in her dotage and could give scarcely any account of herself. She often indulges, her attendant says, who is worn out by her ministrations, loudly in language which is far from the most becoming, and which appears formerly to have been by no means habitual to her.

She has been twice married, lived forty years with her recently deceased husband, and had four children, who are all alive. Had been an industrious, good kind of woman, a spare eater, much more so than now, used to take a little beer or wine, but none latterly, never had any illness so far as the attendant, who had known her well for forty years, is aware; was rather short and thin, but robust, strong and active.

The Rev. F. R. Smith, the curate of Brockdish, informed me that the following are copies from the parish register of Syleham, in Suffolk : "Elizabeth Barber, daughter of George and Sarah Barber, baptized Feb. 1, 1789."—"Elizabeth Barber married to George Duncombe 30th June, 1816."—"Married to Benjamin Atkins Sept. 30th, 1849," the last from the Brockdish register.

Mr Smith remarks that her birthday was always kept on the 6th January, and that it is therefore probable that she was a year old at the time of her baptism, as it is scarcely probable that the ceremony would have taken place when she was only three weeks old. He adds that her niece always heard that she was born in 1787.

Mr Smith further told me that Benjamin Atkins, whose baptism was dated May 11, 1788 [1], was of moderate height, was toothless, had good sight, hearing indifferent ; good appetite and digestion, had been three times married, first to a woman older than himself, on the second occasion to one younger, and

[1] The entry to this effect in the register of the parish church of Bressing is attested by the rector of the parish :—"Benjamin Atkins used to say that he remembered his mother telling him that he was born on Whitsunday. Now in the year 1788 Easter-day was March 23, therefore Whitsunday would be May 11th. If B. A. was not baptized on the day of his birth he must have been a year old on May 11, 1788." F. R. S.

lately to one of the same age; that he used to go about and get up his potatoes till last winter, when he and his wife, as before mentioned, being poor, took to bed as the best mode of keeping themselves warm. A week before his death he took the holy communion, entering heartily into the service. Three days before death his appetite failed; but, with that exception, he seemed well up to the day of his death.

August 22, 1889. I went to-day to Oundle to see Stephen Coal, whose baptismal entry in the vestry of the church I saw, "March 7th, 1787, Stephen son of James and Mary Coal." He had always understood that he was more than six months old when he was baptized; and if that be so he is now at least 103. He is reputed to be 105, and is an inmate of Laxton Hospital, where he has been for 20 or more years. He is a short, small man, about 5 ft. in height, spare and rather bent; enjoys very good health, and has no maladies except a pruriginous skin-eruption on his forearms and arms, which he has had for some time, and which keeps him awake very much at night. He takes salts (half-an-ounce) once or twice a week. He has a remarkably good appetite and digestion, eats more than any other inmate of the hospital, "nothing comes amiss to him and nothing hurts him." His voice is clear and strong, but he hears with one ear only and that imperfectly; is of cheerful, placid disposition; is brisk in his manner and in his answers to questions; goes out every day for short walks, and goes to church on Sundays, often staying for the evening communion. His pulse is between 60 and 70, small and soft, the artery being apparently healthy; but the heart's action is irregular and weak, and there is a distinct systolic bruit heard over its base. Respiration is 20, regular and very gentle, attended with little expansion of the chest, which measures

H. C.   14

about 30 inches, and the walls of which distinctly preserve their elasticity. Scarcely any arcus senilis. One upper molar remains. No evidences of failure in any organ except the heart; and micturition is "very fair."

He was the youngest of five children, has lived in Oundle all his life; was a gardener, therefore much in the open air; led a very regular quiet life, was up early, often at three o'clock fishing; was not a large eater; took about a pint of beer a day, and "occasionally made himself comfortable" when with friends. Never smoked or took snuff. Was never confined to bed by illness. His father lived to 84. His mother died after a confinement. A brother lived to near a hundred, and a sister to over 90. He married at 29 and had six children. A son, æt. 76, who came to see him a few weeks ago, was scarcely as vigorous as himself; and the old man is said to have given "the boy" a penny with which to buy some sweets. There is probably a little mistake as to the age of his son or his own age at the time of his marriage.[1]

The following remarkable statement respecting TWIN CENTENARIANS is quoted in the *Lancet*, August 17, 1889: "On the 12th instant, at Coosat, a village near Athlone, Margaret Mulochill, 100 years of age, gave evidence at a coroner's inquest relative to the death of Honora, her twin sister. The old women lived together, and on Saturday, when Margaret went to the market, she left Honora at home in good health. On returning she found her dead on the sofa. Death had resulted from failure of the heart's action."

The following scarcely less remarkable was a saying, as I am informed by his widow, of the Rev. Mr Williams of Godmanchester: "my Great Aunt sat at the head of her own table for 100 Christmas days; she was married at 15."

[1] He took his daily walk Oct. 10, and died Oct. 12, 1889, after one day's illness.

Post-Mortem Examination (No. 10) of a centenarian.
Professor Cunningham of Trinity College Dublin has
kindly sent me the following account of the Post-Mortem
Examination of "James Conway Æt. 106, born 30th January
1783, died 18th April 1889.

"Dr Kenny who attended him certified his death as being
due to the exhaustion following an acute attack of Cystitis.

"*Appearance of Body.* Well built man of low stature—
spare but muscular. Height 5 ft. 1½ in. Limbs clean and
straight: chest-wall perfectly resilient. *Sternum and Costal
cartilages* showed none of the signs we are in the habit of
associating with old age. Manubrio-gladiolar joint open; no
ossification of costal cartilages.—*Lymphatic glands* in axilla,
groin, chest and mesentery fairly well marked—not enlarged
but certainly not atrophied.—*Heart* small: walls thinner than
usual: still they were firm and the cavities were not dilated.
Valves healthy.—*Lungs* healthy and elastic.—*Intestines* with
thin walls due to atrophy of muscular coat. Peyer's patches
somewhat wasted. In *Stomach* muscular layers better marked.
Liver small, 2 lbs. 1 oz., healthy.—*Spleen* very much reduced
in size.—*Pancreas* very small. (N.B. Spleen, pancreas, and
entire length of injected splenic artery were unfortunately all
weighed together when I was in London. They weighed not
quite 4 oz.)—*Kidneys* and *Suprarenal capsules* normal in
appearance, size and weight.—*Bladder*, muscular coat greatly
hypertrophied.—*Prostate*, size of a small orange and so soft
that it broke down when the capsule was removed in the
dissection of the perineum.—*Cowper's glands* very distinct and
of normal size and appearance.—*Prostatic* and *Vesical plexuses*
of veins not more marked than usual.—*Urethra* wide and
healthy.—*Arteries* throughout the entire body slightly dilated
but with no decided signs of atheroma and little loss of

elasticity.—*Muscles* firm and red—very different from the
oily muscles of my other centenarian [mentioned at p. 103].—
Sigmoid lateral curvature of the spine. This in a measure
accounts for low stature.—*Aorta* showed a corresponding
curvature. The *Brain* was firm and healthy. The cerebral
convolutions were wide apart and somewhat wasted as you
will see [this refers to an excellent model of the head and
brain presented by Prof. Cunningham and placed in the
Museum of the University of Cambridge], and the gaping
fissures were occupied by watery subarachnoid fluid."

The elasticity of the Thorax, the small size of the Spleen
and Peyer's Glands, the healthy condition of the Arteries and
the Costal Cartilages, and the wasted state of the convolutions
of the Brain correspond, on the whole, with the accounts given
(pages 93 to 109) of the nine other examinations of centenarians.
But the Heart is stated to have been small and the Lymphatic
Glands not atrophied.

Prof. Cunningham tells me that this old man never took
alcohol in any form, and did not smoke, that he was an
industrious respectable man who spent a very large part of his
life as a market gardener in the neighbourhood of London;
that he said he had been pressed into the Royal Marines about
1800 and served several years, that he remembered Nelson
well and the story of Lady Hamilton, and that he had scars
of what appeared to be sabre-cuts on his head; Professor
Cunningham adds that the information received from the
Admiralty is that during the period of Nelson's command
there was only one James Conway in the Royal Marines. He
entered the service in 1796 at the age of 18. "Should this be
the Conway in question he must have been 111 and not 106
years of age."

The numerous examples of longevity among the Irish will

probably have been remarked in the preceding pages; and in the *Lancet* Sep. 21 of this year is a notice from the Report of the Registrar General of Ireland (Dr Grimshaw), that the deaths registered during 1888 included no fewer than 208 persons (87 males and 121 females) who were stated to have been aged upwards of one hundred years at the time of their decease. Dr Grimshaw adds that "further inquiry having been made, it was ascertained that the ages of the centenarians as given in the records were in every case confirmed." According to this report the centenarians in Ireland would amount to more than 43 per million of the population, whereas in England and Wales they are estimated at little more than 2 per million. "This" as the *Lancet* adds "is certainly a startling announcement" and needs corroboration. Possibly among the senile, but still quickwitted, Irish the feature of reversion to childhood which loves to exaggerate age may be more strongly developed than it is among the slower inhabit ants on this side the Channel.

Oct. 2, 1889[1], I went to see Mrs Mühlenkemp (*née* Marianne Reed), æt. 100, residing at 35, Markham Square, Chelsea, respecting whom Mr Shield of Chelsea had sent me information. She is a brisk, bright, chatty, withered little woman, "five feet nothing" as she says, with loud clear voice; sight rather failing but able to read a little with glasses which she has used many years; much arcus senilis; rather deaf; joints of hand natural; scarcely remembers having any teeth; moderate appetite and digestion; takes about an ounce of meat daily and a little wine or whiskey at night; regular action of bowels, rarely taking medicine; very energetic and intelligent and with excellent memory; has not been out of the house for

---

[1] This makes the *seventy-fourth* centenarian of whom an account has been given in this book.

two years, but walks a little about the house; goes to bed about six and gets up after breakfast; does not sleep very well, thinking and pondering a good deal at night; has no malady but feels weak and short-breathed; her respiration is 36 and there is a little bronchial trouble, but the sounds of the heart are natural, and the pulse is 80, regular, rather firm, without any knottiness of the artery. She is troubled a little with incontinence of urine.

She was the seventh of a family of ten, was born Sept. 10th, 1789, in London[1] and has lived there the chief part of her life; was married at 20; her husband lived 50 years but she had no children; was always spare ("They used to call her the fairy"), and had good health and digestion; was a small eater, took very little meat and no beer or wine or spirit till lately, very active, an early riser and good sleeper. She broke her wrist sliding on the ice when young and her arm by a fall at 96 which united, Mr Shield says, very quickly. Her only illness was an attack of obstruction of the bowels ten years ago. Her father died at the age of 78, her mother at 70. "Most of her brothers and sisters lived into the seventies."

Lord Byron, when about 12, lodged with his mother at a tailor's in Half Moon St. next door to where she lived, and was very fond of her. The children used to play together. He was a good playmate but bad-tempered; and he and his mother quarrelled so much that the lodging-house people would not keep them. He went to Harrow and she saw no more of him. Several of the French refugee nobles lodged at her mother's house. Her husband was a Hanoverian, and

[1] She says that she was baptised in St George's Church, Hanover Square; and the following is the extract from the Register Book of Baptisms of that Parish:
"Sep. 25 1789 Mary Anne Daughter of Joseph & Ann Reed, born Sep. 10."
She states that Joseph and Ann were the names of her father and mother

escaped to England when Napoleon entered his native town; was in the service of the Duke of Kent and much patronised by him. He acted as courier to various young noblemen; and she travelled over great part of the Continent with him. Subsequently he was made principal door-keeper at the House of Lords; and she there became acquainted with many of the members of that house. The Duke of Wellington told her "she was the cleverest little body in the House." At the time of the fire at the Houses of Parliament she knew where the mace was to be found and was the means of saving it. She does not "much care whether her life is further prolonged or not." It is to be hoped that she may have that tranquil easy departure which is commonly accorded to those who have lived so long.

ILLUSTRATIONS.

FRONTISPIECE: Photograph of Benjamin Atkins and his wife, each of whom was 101 (see page 208).

Of the following PHOTOGRAPHS the first shows the section of the Upper End of the Thigh-bone of an adult man, the form of the part, the angle of the neck with the shaft, and the structure of the interior. The wall of the bone, enclosing the medullary cavity, is seen to be thick below, to diminish in thickness as it ascends into the neck in consequence of plates separating from it which form the cancelli of the neck, head and great trochanter. A vertical series of these cancelli ascend to the uppermost part of the head; they are the chief recipients of weight from the pelvis, and serve to transmit the weight from that part to the inner side of the wall of the shaft. Others form an arch subtending the upper wall of the neck and transmitting weight from it to both sides of the wall of the shaft.

The second shows a similar section from a woman reported to have died at the age of 103. There is no reduction in the size or alteration in the form of the bone. Indeed, for a woman, it is large, and the neck forms an open angle with its shaft. But it contrasts with No. 1 remarkably in the thinness of the wall of the bone, which has resulted from absorption at the interior, and in the diminution of the cancelli with the consequent enlargement of the spaces between them. The bony plates which form the arch subtending the upper wall of the neck can scarcely be recognised, and the vertical series ascending to the summit of the head are much reduced in number and size.

The contrast thus presented is sufficient to account for the fact that fracture in this region is common in old persons—especially in women, the angle of the neck with the shaft being at all periods of life more open in women than in men—though it is comparatively rare in adults and young persons.

The LITHOGRAPH-PLATE represents the Lower Jaw-bone at different periods of life:

Fig. 1, at birth, when the angle is wide, the neck being nearly in a line with the body of the bone, which chiefly consists of the alveolary, or tooth-socket, part. The dental canal and the mental hole, which transmit the nerve to the teeth and the lower lip, are near the lower edge of the bone.

Fig. 2 represents the jaw at about the third year. The neck is still nearly in a line with the body of the bone, and the sockets for the teeth (of the first and second dentition) still occupy a considerable part of its thickness.

Fig. 3 is the massive jaw of an adult, in which the neck, or rather the ascending portion that carries the neck, is nearly at a right angle with the body of the bone. The latter is chiefly formed by, and derives its strength chiefly from, the *sub*-alveolary part. The mental hole is at a considerable distance from the lower edge.

Fig. 4 is the jaw of an old person, apparently an old woman. It resembles the infantile jaw in the obliquity of its ascending part, but quite differs from it in that the alveolary or dental portion has disappeared and the *sub*-dental part only of the body of the bone remains. The mental hole, indicated by a bristle, is on the upper edge.

Fig. 5 represents the facial bones of an old person. The alveolary parts of both upper and lower jaws are quite gone. The obliquity of the neck and ascending portion of the lower jaw throws the mental part far in front of the upper jaw, and brings the chin and nose, supposing the projecting soft part of the latter to be present, into very near proximity.

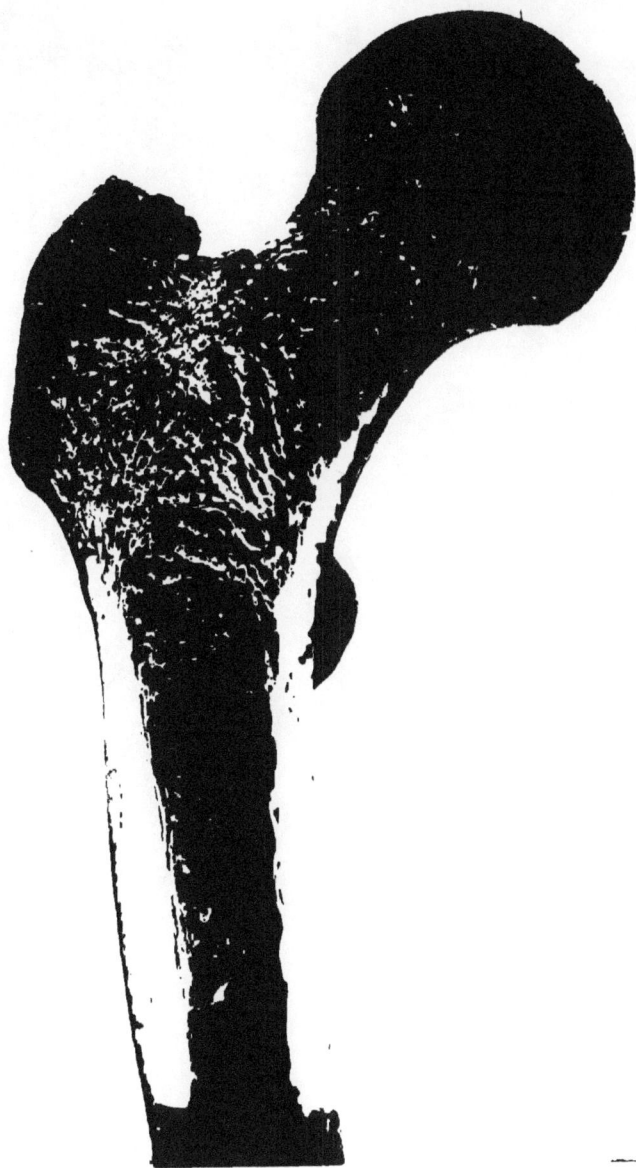

2.—INTERIOR OF UPPER END OF ADULT THIGH-BONE.

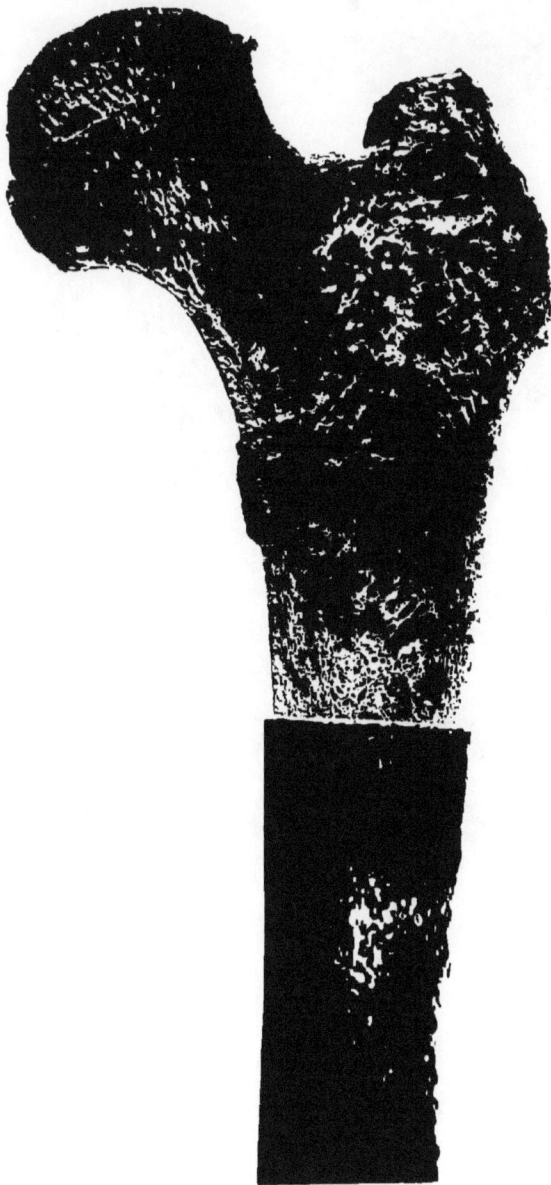

Permanent Photo.

Colin Lunn, Cambridge.

3.—INTERIOR OF UPPER END OF THIGH-BONE ÆT 103.

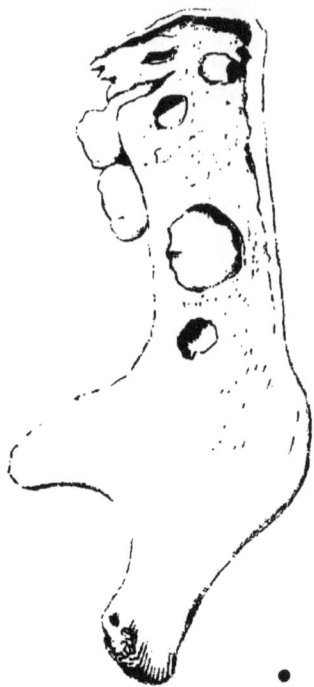

2. Third year

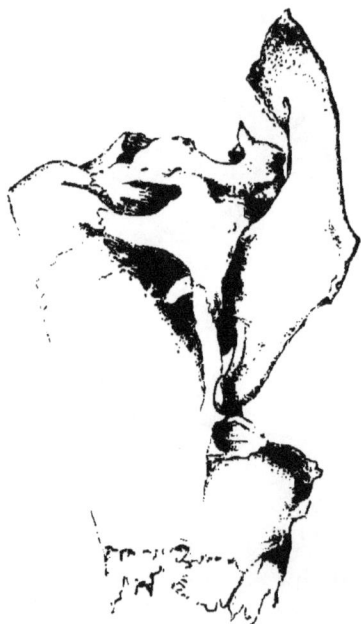

5. Senile, reduced

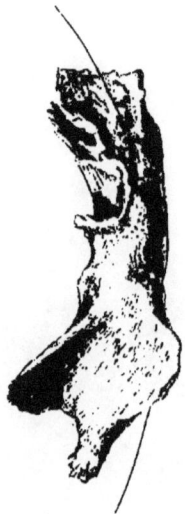

1. At birth

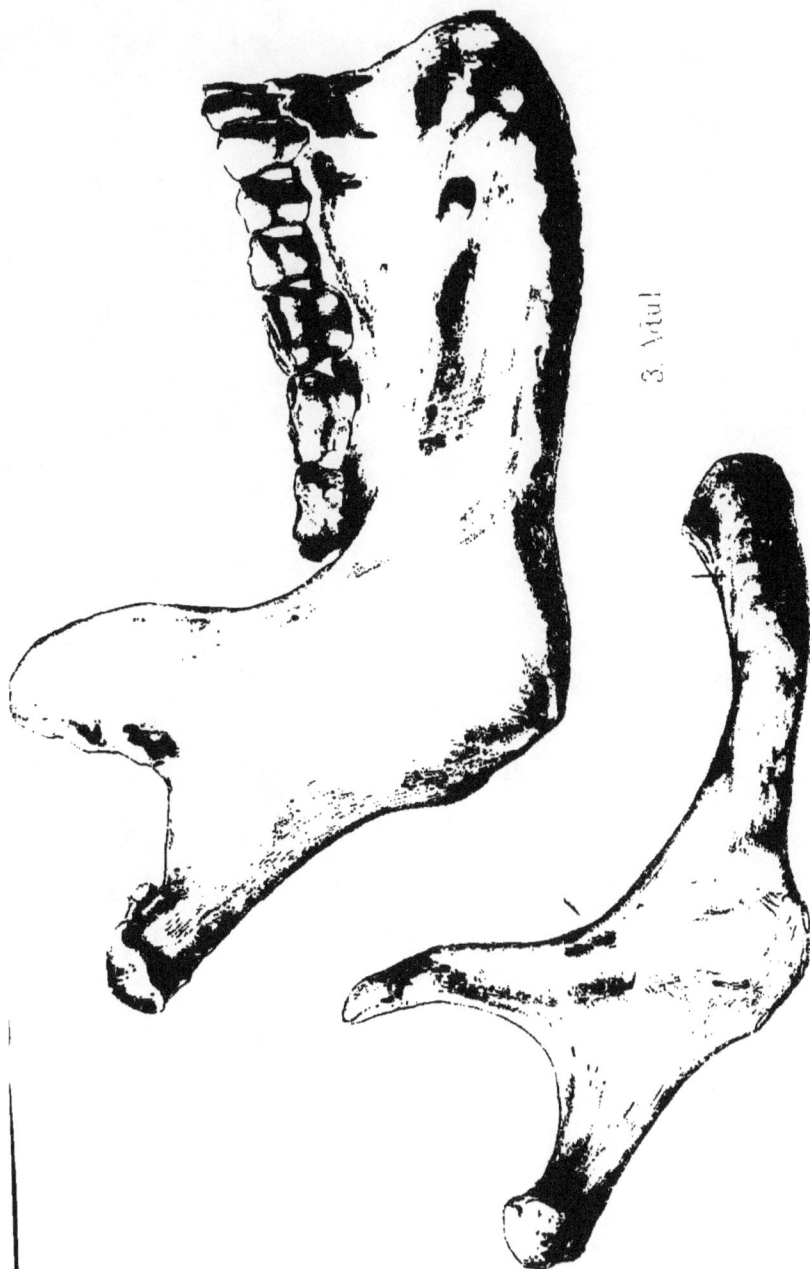

3. Adult

INDEX.

H. C.   15

CAMBRIDGE: PRINTED BY C. J. CLAY, M.A. AND SONS, AT THE UNIVERSITY PRESS.

www.ingramcontent.com/pod-product-compliance
Lightning Source LLC
Chambersburg PA
CBHW030733280326
41926CB00086B/1302